THE ENDURING
EFFECTS OF
PRENATAL EXPERIENCE

THE ENDURING EFFECTS OF PRENATAL EXPERIENCE

ECHOES FROM THE WOMB

Dr. Ludwig Janus

**Translated by
Terence Dowling**

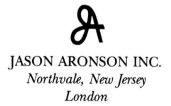

JASON ARONSON INC.
Northvale, New Jersey
London

This book was set in 11 pt. New Baskerville by Alabama Book Composition of Deatsville, Alabama and printed and bound by Book-mart Press of North Bergen, New Jersey.

Library of Congress Cataloging-in-Publication Data

Janus, Ludwig, 1939–
    [Wie die Seele entsteht.   English]
    The enduring effects of prenatal experience : echoes from the womb / by Ludwig Janus.
        p.   cm.
    Includes bibliographical references and index.
    ISBN 1-56821-853-2 (h/c : alk. paper)
        1. Infants (Newborn) — Psychology.   2. Childbirth — Psychological aspects.   3. Behavioral embryology.   I. Title.
    BF719.J3613   1997
    152.42′2 — dc20   96-17634

This book was originally published in German in 1991 by Hoffmann und Campe Verlag, Hamburg. Copyright © 1991 by Hoffmann und Campe.

Printed in the United States of America on acid-free paper. Jason Aronson Inc. offers books and cassettes. For information and catalog write to Jason Aronson Inc., 230 Livingston Street, Northvale, New Jersey 07647. Or visit our website: http://www.aronson.com

Dedicated to my wife and family

Contents

Introduction

One of the first big questions that a child asks is about where babies come from. The answer the parents give is crucial for the child's understanding of himself. And, as we all know, the answer is almost always unsatisfactory. Whereas in earlier times recourse was made to fairy tales or mythical powers, that, for example, the child had been delivered by a stork or had grown from a tree, nowadays, in keeping with the scientific spirit of the times, most people try to describe our coming to the light of day in purely biological or physical terms. All questions about the possible significance of the experience of being born are left unasked and unanswered. Thus, even the stories that portray birth as a journey, an adventure or a transition from one world to another, are more revealing. Children and adults remain more or less untouched by the statement that babies come from mothers' bellies. Any personally significant question is thereby simply avoided and one is left with the feeling that something unknown is lurking just around the corner.

What is the significance of spending nine months in the secret recesses of a woman's body? What did I sense and feel and experience there? To most in our modern culture, such questions still seem quite inappropriate, only things a child could ask. However, now, toward the end of this millennium, serious questions about the significance of birth, of our having been born, are being asked.

The first major breakthroughs with regard to the question "Is my birth significant for me?" were made in the pioneer works of psychoanalysts Otto Rank and Hans Gustav Graber, which appeared in 1924. Both of these men realized that birth is experienced and that this first experience of "coming into the world" provides a fundamental pattern for our future experiencing and development. One can often see this background pattern clearly in the feelings of mentally unstable patients but also in various cultural phenomena. A fear of darkness or claustrophobia can be the echo of an individual's traumatic birth experience just as much as the need that groups have to come together in special, safe places can be rooted in a longing for the original security of our first uterine home.

At first glance, such connections seem to go against common sense. And indeed, that such statements can be made with any plausibility at all requires the careful synthesis of various strands of modern research. "Prenatal psychology" is the umbrella title for the endeavors that unite various scientific disciplines in their attempt to elucidate the processes of experience involved in the earliest stages of human life.

Although it is now a generally accepted matter of fact that the child we once were continues to live on in the adult we have become, it is still quite strange for us to see the baby or the unborn child that we also once were in the same way.

This idea is challenging in a way not dissimilar to the challenge brought about by developments in the last decades in the field of human ethology. The parallel is instructive. Konrad Lorenz and his followers have shown that Darwin's theory—that humans evolved out of the animal kingdom—is to be understood as the evolution not only of external characteristics but also of internal mechanisms of behavior. Animals are in fact much closer relatives than we normally care to admit, which remains extremely difficult for us to recognize within ourselves and to accept any similarities. We have a similar difficulty when it comes to recognizing a much closer relative, namely, the unborn child or the newborn baby within ourselves. We have to sacrifice a little of the security that a purely postnatal view of our existence fosters and at the same time allow ourselves to be confronted with such elementary feelings as those of dependence, helplessness, and panic, which are so often present during birth.

This book offers an introduction to the recent developments in the psychology of birth and of human life before birth. In so doing, it also opens the reader to an understanding of his or her own birth and the significance of his or her own experience of having been born. However, it must not be forgotten that the very fact that the book could be written at all is evidence of a fundamental shift in present day attempts to understand ourselves. It could not have been written fifty years ago and no doubt completely different horizons will open up within the next twenty years. This shift has been especially impressed upon me in my work as a psychotherapist, in which access to birth memories and to prenatal stages of experience has now become common-place. However, as will be shown in detail, approaches to these questions have been developed within many different disciplines. Full use will be made of quotations in order to communicate these new developments.

However, the emotional difficulties involved in attempt-ing to approach birth and prenatal life in a personal way should not be underestimated. In the first place, birth is for us humans relatively traumatic. This is due to the biological facts of our upright posture and our relatively large brain. Both of these evolutionary developments have necessitated that humans be born earlier than otherwise would be good for them. Thus the adventure and exhilaration of coming into the world is regularly accompanied by a mixture of uncertainty, desperate aggression, and even fear of annihi-lation.

Thus, parallel to the fascination that the subject of birth and life before birth awakens within us, there is an even stronger diffidence and diffuse reluctance to look closer and examine our deep emotions. Many readers will almost certainly experience this difficulty. Despite all of the advan-tageous developments in obstetric practice in this century, the purely medical-technological approach that governs modern maternity clinics does not prevent all sorts of psychological trauma from being inflicted upon us during and shortly after birth. The simple statement of this quite obvious fact is itself enough to elicit an uncanny feeling of resistance in most people.

The second important difficulty that arises as soon as we try to understand the earliest stages of life is that we don't have the same access to our birth and life in the womb that we do to subsequent early experiences—say, for example, to the experience of starting nursery school. In fact, it is now recognized that much of our early experience is revealed and concealed in fairy tales about other worlds, in mythology, and in our religious imaginings. Belief in the well-being and security that an almighty being can guarantee or in a social utopia of a heavenly kingdom on earth can express the wish to return to a prenatal paradise. The fear rooted in prenatal panic can express itself in fantasies of hell and eternal punishment.

Both of the above-mentioned difficulties have led to a third problem, namely the denial of any connection between the earliest stages of life and those that follow. There was a shift in this denial at the beginning of our century with the acceptance of the discovery that childhood experiences— still excluding the very earliest ones—are of significance for later development. Before this shift, the rejection of childhood was demonstrated clearly in the ways in which parents could treat their children with full social and legal acceptance. Babies were given away, sold, or killed, or if kept were cared for by paid staff or strangers. All of this is rightly condemned today. However, we still remain estranged from the very small baby within us and unquestioningly rely on external norms and authorities to determine what happens to our newborn and unborn children. As long as we deny any personal awareness of our life before birth, of our birth, and of earliest baby years, and as long as we repress the significance of early experience for a fuller understanding of human life, then we are also condemned to distancing ourselves emotionally from our unborn and newborn offspring. The next generation then remains unprotected from blind repetition of the same mishandling and traumata that lie buried but quite alive and active within our unconscious minds.

The last few decades have witnessed the beginnings of a relaxation of this deepest area of denial. This can be recognized above all in the "gentle birth" movement and in the recognition of the significance of the earliest traumata in various schools of psychotherapy (for example, in primal therapy). It can also be seen in the growing number of empirical studies of pre- , peri- , and postnatal processes of perception and behavior. Indeed, this new climate alone has allowed the research and development of our theme: the personal, biographical significance of our existence before birth and of the process of our birth. However, the previous tradition of denial of prenatal human existence has not yet been fully transcended and we all still live more or less under its influence.

We are still exposed to countless prejudices—for example, that the unborn and newborn baby are insensitive and unconscious, with no memory abilities. Only further research leading to a better knowledge of the earliest stages of human psychological life—before, during, and after birth—can lead to a new and deeper understanding of ourselves, to a better start in life for our children, and to a better world.

1

"The Bundle of Life" and Superstition During Pregnancy: Prelude to Prenatal Psychology

Each individual culture symbolizes and explores prenatal experience and its significance for later development in quite different ways. As mentioned in the introduction, many traces of pre- and perinatal events are preserved in mythological stories and in rites of passage. The baby's experience of its own placenta is expressed explicitly in stories in which the placenta is described as brother, guardian spirit, or source of power (see "Nachgeburt" in Bächtold-Stäubli 1987a, Davidson 1985).

Several thousand years ago in the high culture of Egypt, elements of prenatal life were built into official state ceremony in a uniquely concrete and at the same time symbolic way. The placenta, which had sustained the Pharaoh, was a most significant and respected object (Frankfort 1942). It was preserved in a container and there was an official called "Opener of the Royal Placenta." As a symbol of security, the placenta was carried as a standard in processions. Furthermore, there were also the so-called life bundles, which contained the placenta and were ceremonially opened at the end of the king's reign (Murray 1930). These facts are of significance for an understanding of the development of the human religious imagination because the hieroglyph for the life bundle later became the sign for the Egyptian concept of God.

A primitive awareness of prenatal existence expressed itself not only in religious myth and ritual but also in a more or less explicit teaching about the psychological life of the unborn child. In India, for example, there are traditions for the "care of the embryonal soul of the developing child." The Indian psychoanalyst Sudhir Kakar (1984) writes:

At birth and the cutting of the umbilical cord, the connection . . . to cosmic consciousness . . . is interrupted. A hole appears in the area around the navel. . . . The well-known "navel-gazing" in the East is literally the contemplation of this hole, which . . . in Hindu thought is called "Maya" and which separates the individual's consciousness from its universal roots. [p. 207]

It is also quite remarkable with what openness and ease the Indonesians fantasize about the events of pregnancy in their literature. The psychotherapist Helga Blazy (1991a) who understands the East Asiatic mentality very well, writes: "The Indonesian culture and its literature have an advantage over the West in that they know no break and no taboo between conception, pregnancy and life outside of the womb. For them, being and life does not suddenly begin at birth" (p. 163).

Quite differently from in Western cultures, the child is also recognized before its birth in China and Japan. Then when it appears at birth, it is considered to be already 1 year old. Another impressive example of openness toward unborn human life is to be found in the Mbuti, an African tribe that the ethnologist Colin Turnbull (1983) has described in a quite moving way. (Further examples are described by Gupta and Gupta 1989, Hakanson 1988, and Kilbridge 1990.)

Until the eighteenth century in our culture, people's practical approach to prenatal psychology was influenced by the idea that mistakes made by the mother were significant. Folk belief held that strong emotional experiences, imaginings, and worries of the mother could have an effect on her unborn child. They could be the cause, on the one hand, of physical things such as birthmarks and, on the other, of character traits. In fact, folk belief understood the result of such prenatal influences to be quite direct:

> If the pregnant woman makes a slip with a tight rope walker, then the child develops dangly arms and legs and cannot walk or stand. If the mother makes a mistake in being frightened by a mouse or a dog, then the child gets micy skin or a dog's foot as a result; if by a hare, then the child gets a trembling chin or a hare-lip. Being shocked by a mouse or a frog gives the child a protuberance or a birthmark which looks like that animal. [Bächtold-Stäubli 1987b, p. 1422]

According to the theory, the cravings of the pregnant woman are also significant. The superstition recommends that "the cravings should be complied with wholeheartedly and the woman should be in no way refused. . . . In Schlesia they believe that psoriasis is caused by stopping a pregnant woman from craving after fish" (Bächtold-Stäubli 1987a, p. 1417).

In the eighteenth century, there was a lively debate about this theory and the supporters of the idea went on the defensive. The rational-positivist mentality that ruled natural science of the day made any discussion about human psychological life before birth out of the question. Nevertheless, with the transition to romanticism, proponents of the "blunder theory" managed to popularize several ideas full of insight. Thus, for example, the Swiss theologian and author Johann Kaspar Lavater (1741–1801) wrote:

> If a woman could keep an accurate record of the various strong imaginings which crossed her mind during the pregnancy, she would then perhaps be able to perceive the philosophical, moral, intellectual and physiognomic destiny of her child in advance. [quoted in Bennholdt-Thomsen and Guzzoni 1990, p. 116]

Quite realistically, the educationalist Joachim Heinrich Campe (1746–1818) saw in the normal conditions of pregnancy "a fatal lesson in suffering" for the unborn child. The novelist, nowadays hardly known, who wrote *Sturm und Drang* (Storm and Urge), Johann Karl Wezel (1747–1819) wrote:

> It has been realised that, if not all, then most of the phenomena, which to the consternation of learned and simple alike can be observed in many people and which remain at present unexplained, that these can be understood quite easily if one makes known the exact and detailed history of their fate in the womb from the first moment of their

existence up until after their birth. [quoted in Bennholdt-Thomsen and Guzzoni 1990, p. 117]

Such prenatal psychological associations were in fact made as early as 1738 in Adam Berns's autobiography. He writes:

All of which [the war situation] made her terribly frightened, so that it is not to be wondered that she brought into the world a melancholic (child) with a constricted heart, one which the mother had carried for nine months under a contrite heart oppressed by fear and dread; *partus enim sequitor conditionem ventris* [for the departed (child) is followed by the conditions of the womb]. [quoted in Bennholdt-Thomsen and Guzzoni 1990, p. 117]

In E. T. A. Hoffman's (1967) famous novel, *The Woman from Scuderi*, a direct connection is made between the prenatal experience of the main character and his later life. A prenatal trauma rooted in the mother's confrontation with death and her mania for jewels during the pregnancy becomes the hero's fate and is permanently repeated in his own sick passion for jewels and in the murders and thefts that he commits.

However, the insights and intuition of a few individuals into the deep roots of our psyche did not lead to a general acceptance and understanding of human prenatal existence but were lost and forgotten. The apodictic statement of the French psychologist and educationalist Jules Gabriel Compayré (1843–1913) in his book *The Development of the Child's Psyche* (1900) is a good example of this tendency. For him, psychological life begins only after birth. He deals rigorously with the French authors of the seventeenth century like Nicolas Malebranche who had accepted the fact of human life before birth. Malebranche (1674) assumed that there was an internal connection between the deep experience of the child and that of the mother, while Pierre-Jean-Georges Cabanis (1757–1808) thought that, because the unborn child possessed senses, it must also have a rudimentary psychological life before birth.

Even in the middle of the twentieth century, the medical world, when not downright negative, tended to be very reticent about the possibility of prenatal experience. Until quite recently, surgery was carried out on newborn babies without anesthetic because they were denied psychological life and pain sensitivity! This practice was only changed after increased stress hormone levels had been measured in babies being operated on without anesthetic (Anand and Hickey 1982, Brosch and Rust 1989).

While the nineteenth century attitude toward prenatal life was preserved in the traditions of school medicine, the development of psychoanalysis and of modern art marked the onset of a new approach. Because Freud emphasized the importance of childhood experience and the extreme psychological sensitivity of the child, he initiated a complete turnaround in perspective. From then on early experience was seen to be intrusive and formative, very often bordering on traumatic; later experiences build upon early ones and, because of more developed psychological capabilities, are much easier to handle. However, Freud was unwilling to develop his ideas about the effects of early experience through to their logical conclusion. It was a midwife who was eventually able to convince him that a child experiences fear during its birth:

It may perhaps interest you to learn how anyone could have formed such an idea as that the act of birth is the source and prototype of the affect of anxiety. Speculation had a very small share in it; what I did, rather, was to borrow from the naïve popular mind. Long years ago, while I was sitting with a number of other young hospital doctors at our mid-day meal in an inn, a house physician from the midwifery department told us of a comic thing that had happened at the last examination for midwives. A candidate was asked what it meant if meconium (excreta) made its appearance at birth in the water coming away, and she promptly replied: 'it means the child's frightened.' She was laughed at and failed in the examination. But silently I took her side and began to suspect that this poor woman from the humbler classes had laid an unerring finger on an important correlation. [Freud 1966b, p. 412]

The Hungarian psychoanalyst Sandor Ferenczi (1964a) later traced the significance of good prenatal conditions. He described them as providing the model for feelings of omnipotence and good fortune. It was his impression that the newborn baby to some extent grieved for his prenatal life:

When one observes the general behaviour of the newborn child, one gains the impression that it was not constructed for the harsh disturbance of that perfect peace it enjoyed in its mother's womb and that it longs to return to its previous condition. All who tend to babies instinctively recognize this desire. As soon as a child shows its listlessness by wriggling and screaming, they purposely bring it into a position which resembles being in the womb as much as possible. They lie it on the mother's warm body or wrap it in soft, warm blankets and padding—obviously to create for it the illusion of the mother's protective warmth. They protect its eyes from light, its ears from loud noise and make it possible for it to continue to enjoy intrauterine bliss; or they reproduce the soft, rhythmic, monotonous stimuli which the child even in utero cannot avoid (the rocking movements as the mother walks around, the maternal heart beat, the dull noises from the surroundings which reach the body's insides) by rocking the baby and by softly humming monotonous, rhythmic lullabies. [p. 68]

Ferenczi understood the psychological life of the newborn as being essentially influenced by a hallucinatory desire to restore the satisfying conditions of undisturbed existence in the warm and peaceful womb. The strength of this desire, which is above all to be seen in the symbolic creations of neurotically sick children and adults, was explained by the psychoanalyst Otto Rank as rooted in birth, an experience that due to human evolution is unavoidably traumatic. It is this that in turn determines the intensity of the desire to return to the previous good condition, a desire that can manifest itself in an infinite number of symbols and foundational motifs in human psychology.

At the beginning of the 1920s, the pioneer work of obstetricians such as Philip Schwartz (1966) and Hans Saenger (1924), among others, who had recognized the traumatic aspect of birth on the physical level seemed to confirm the conclusions of Otto Rank. However, the work of Rank and Schwartz stirred up such deep feelings, resistance, and disquiet that the scientific interest in the subject again receded for a while. In the following years, some courageous individuals pursued research into the continuity of human experience from prenatal to postnatal life. This research has been intensified especially in the last twenty years, resulting in more scientific congresses and the appearance of more publications on the subject. This newfound knowledge now facilitates a comprehensive presentation. One precondition for the study of the special aspects of human birth, however, is an understanding of evolutionary factors, which will be discussed in the next chapter.

2

Always a Trauma? The Evolutionary Development of Human Birth

EVOLUTIONARY FACTORS

Whereas the sea offers an expansive environment in which young marine animals can grow from the very beginning of their life onward, creatures on land must protect their very young from the danger of drying out by providing a very special milieu. In the course of evolution, the animals that could fly developed the relatively safe and protective system of the egg in which to contain their embryos, that is, a place outside of the mother's body. The mother bird would be too handicapped in her flying if she had to carry her babies with her. It is therefore very advantageous for her to lay eggs. However, during the embryonic phase of a young bird's life, its temperature regulation is almost completely dependent on the brooding of the parents. Then, the rigidity of the eggshell forces the baby birds to emerge in a relatively immature condition. They are not completely developed and must remain in a second protective place, the nest, and be fed by the parent birds until they reach maturity.

None of the above considerations apply to nonflying land animals. For the mammals, the development of a protective compartment inside the mother's body proved to be successful. The protection that the mammalian parents could offer in this way was not as limited as that of the birds. The length of time that the baby can stay inside its mother can simply be increased until the baby has developed enough to survive in the external environment. So, for example, pregnancy in elephants lasts twenty months. As a result, practically all mammals are so well developed by the time of their birth that they do not need any nest and can more or less immediately cope in the adult animals' world.

The evolution of human birth has been complicated by the need to respond to a number of different demands. The progressive development of the brain and the accompanying increase in the volume of the skull demanded an enlargement of the birth canal in humans. However, the development of the upright position required a narrower and rigid pelvic bone, with an indentation caused by the S-shaped spinal column. Only this S-form column could carry the weight of the upright body. The evolutionary solution to this dilemma was to halve the length of the human pregnancy. The peculiar helplessness of human babies in the first year of their life is a direct result of this fact. One can thus speak of this first year of life as the "extrauterine premature year" of human development (Portmann 1969).

The changes in the pelvis due to the upright posture

produced a bend in the birth canal. Furthermore, the upper opening is oval from side to side while below the pelvis is oval from back to front. The child must therefore make a turn of 90 degrees during the process of birth, and an axial distortion of the neck results from this. This in turn leads to the development of a so-called locus minoris resistentia (a weak point) at this point in the neck because the spine with such a twist cannot cope with the labor contractions so well. In addition, the spinal arteries are also bent and the blood supply to the brain is impeded. The narrowness of the birth canal necessitates that humans cannot be born like their nearest relatives with an intact amnion to cushion the pressure of the contractions. Instead of that, during the last phase of the birth, the full pressure is delivered to the child's head, which becomes deformed. This leads to the so-called compound displacement of the child's brain (Müller 1973). In comparison to our nearest relatives, the apes, the human birth canal is much narrower and convoluted. But fetal growth in humans is much quicker so that the newborn is comparatively bigger. This makes human birth much more difficult than that of apes, and, above all, it takes considerably longer (see de Snoo 1942, Kurrek 1986, Müller 1990a,b, Naaktgeboren and Slijper 1986).

From the evolutionary point of view, it is quite clear that human birth is a relatively novel phenomenon, the end product of a complex power struggle between several biological requirements. The calamity of human birth is the result (Kurrek 1988, Müller 1991). Our birth canal passes through the one solid ring of bone in the body, that ring which in man's egg-laying ancestors previously served to protect the egg (Riedl 1985). This route was so fixed in nature's blueprint that it could not be bypassed in later evolutionary developments.

It can be taken for granted that the true complexity of this situation has not yet been fully understood. Recent research has highlighted another important factor: birth occurs when the placenta can no longer supply enough oxygen to the baby (Prechtl 1987). It is in any case probable that, in comparison to apes, the rapid increase in weight during the human fetal period is itself an attempt to compensate for the vulnerability caused by the baby's being born too early. This early birth makes human newborns very sensitive to temperature. Thus, as a protection against later cold, human fetuses develop a thick fat tissue under their skin, a development that does not occur in other primates but that in humans makes up for 16 percent of the body weight (Schachtinger 1987). This also represents a further burden upon the mother and limits the possible length of pregnancy.

SOCIAL FACTORS

The complexity of the evolutionary factors that have determined the beginning of human life can also be seen in the fact that our premature birth is only possible when combined with a change in instinctive, social behavior, especially of the mother but also of the family and extended social group (Trevathan 1990). The parents must be prepared to form a sort of social womb so that their child can survive despite its being born prematurely. The picture of the unborn baby secure in its mother's womb tends to disguise the fact that the individual who has appeared from the fertilized egg is from the very beginning a unique living being with enormous developmental potential and possibility of reaction. During the various developmental phases of prenatal existence, that individual regulates itself and its relationship to its environment in a variety of ways.

Observation of prematurely born babies has made it abundantly clear that sense perception, emotional reaction, and motor response develop very rapidly before birth. Because these babies, who have left the protection of their mother's womb too soon, are completely dependent on emotional and physical closeness in order to survive and develop, it can be taken for granted that the unborn child also experiences an intimate, emotional bond to its mother. One can observe with ultrasound how an unborn child will react with interest to an emotionally warm approach but moves away from anything repellent.

PSYCHOLOGICAL FACTORS

The above observations give an idea of the psychological consequences of the evolutionary peculiarities of human birth. Because of our premature birth, humans are not only physically but even more so psychologically ill-prepared to face postnatal life. Only a continuous bonding to the mother or an adequate substitute and the development of a relationship of marked dependence on her, accompanied by all the appropriate emotions, can compensate for our immaturity as newborns. It is quite plausible to claim that this elementary feeling of dependence is reflected in religious beliefs in a merciful, almighty, and loving Being, and that these beliefs in turn provide us with a vivid picture of what the infant experiences. As with all other physical, perceptual, and psychological functions, we must assume that this dependence also begins to develop prenatally. If it were not present before birth, it just could not be available so readily after birth. These, then, are the reasons for the extreme sensitivity of human babies to all forms of stress and their proneness to feelings of insecurity. Human newborn survival is only certain when the baby reacts promptly to insecurity and discomfort with vigorous crying.

But even before birth, babies react to disturbances of all kinds by rash movements and facial expressions of discomfort. They can also be heard crying when air has happened to enter the uterus, for example, during a medical examination (Liley and Day 1967, Ryder 1943). To hear this crying of the unborn child is one of the most moving experiences that can occur in connection with pregnancy. The unborn human person can suddenly no longer be avoided. Apart from noticing strong movements inside their bellies, pregnant mothers generally perceive their child's emotional reactions and impulses only in a very limited way. As a result, it is quite possible that the mother–fetus relationship is inadequately protected. Especially in our complex culture with its many demands, there is even an increased danger that the mother leaves herself and her unborn child open to too much psychological and physical stress. The child is just too hidden from view in the womb.

During the past few decades in our Western culture, we have developed a deeper understanding of the special sensitivity and vulnerability of the infant. A similar understanding for unborn human life is just beginning.

TRAUMATIC CONSEQUENCES

Whoever hears the evolutionary facts about human birth will fear that it is fundamentally flawed and in principle traumatic. Unfortunately, the studies of various obstetricians have confirmed this fear. Postmortems of children who died during or shortly after birth have shown a frighteningly high incidence of hemorrhage and damage to the brain, even in children who showed no other signs of trauma. Also, modern techniques like computed tomography have shown that damage to the child's brain occurs far more frequently than previously accepted. Sadly we must presume that the only conclusion to be drawn from this information about organic damage is that birth, also in its psychological aspects, is generally traumatic. This trauma leads to feelings of fear, panic, anger, despair, and shame, and feelings of total shock and annihilation, as if one were being torn apart.

The more or less massive psychological destruction that occurs at birth can, when it is not understood and compensated for in an accepting and caring relationship, lead to further stress in the early mother–child relationship and even prevent a good relationship from developing in the first place. Thus all efforts to secure "gentle birth" in our societies are of fundamental importance. Social and cultural demands that are not easy to harmonize with our instincts have also had terrible effects on our birth practices. Only a deeper knowledge of all the factors involved can help us to prevent avoidable damage.

POSITIVE EFFECTS OF THE BIRTH PROCESS

In stark contrast to all these dangers that our premature birth as humans brings with it, there is perhaps also a special advantage for our further development. Birth represents a remarkable achievement and to have succeeded in this challenging transition at the beginning of our postnatal existence possibly prepares us to strive with the same effort in all later struggles. All later transitions, for example that of becoming an adult or even of death itself, can be understood and managed as new births. It is also possible that the extreme dependence so characteristic of humans during their prenatal and early postnatal life is the origin of our ability to sacrifice the self and to be committed to one goal. Both of these abilities are absolutely fundamental for the development of human culture.

To understand the psychological significance of our birth experience better, it is necessary to consider the fact that we cannot ourselves remember the very earliest phases of our life. This problem, the so-called early childhood amnesia, is the subject of the next chapter.

3

"But I Can't Remember . . .": The Problem of Early Childhood Amnesia

Many people have difficulty remembering events in their childhood. Their memory fails for events prior to the age of 10. This is often the case when the family was full of conflict and difficulty and did not always foster a strong sense of identity throughout the various phases of the child's development. Adult lack of empathy for and lack of interest in their children, such as the practice that was not so long ago very common of letting babies cry, and the frequent beating of small children, can only happen if adults are estranged from their own childhood. In many biographies from previous times, childhood is presented only in very hazy and idealized terms, almost as something strange and foreign.

Modern psychological knowledge and insight into everyday life has produced a great change here. Nowadays many people strive for a realistic picture of their own childhood and a better relationship to the child still within them. The decrease in social repression in general and the better awareness of bodily functions, which has been developing slowly since the beginning of the twentieth century, have helped further this goal. As a result, questions about the significance of early childhood amnesia can now be handled differently. We are much more used to the idea that childhood experience lives on not only in our memories but in our emotional attitudes, our hopes, our expectations, and our convictions.

PREVERBAL MEMORIES

Psychologists and doctors have various opinions about preverbal memories. With the acquisition of language, the child's ego is extended and this extension forms the basis for the development of our self-reflective identity. Preverbal experiences are thus not like the later self-centered ones. Rather they have an holistic character. Here is an example:

> A student experienced a lot of fear while she had a bout of fever and imagined that something was moving in big circles around her face. The circles got smaller and the thing began to move faster until something suddenly darted towards her with a loud, buzzing noise and she began to scream. When the mother heard about her daughter's fear, she said: "I kept telling your father not to do it." Apparently the father had tried to get a reaction from the baby when she was only a few days old in the following way: he stood in front of her cot and moved his hand in front of the baby's face, at first making big

circles followed by quicker and smaller ones. The whole performance ended when he suddenly made a hissing noise and tickled the child under the chin. The mother had observed that the child got an emotional shock every time and had told the father so. [Kruse 1969, p. 74]

This is a typical example of the way in which an early experience can be remembered. The whole experience is repeated, and the past becomes a present event. It does not become a memory that one can reflect on in a more or less uninvolved way. Positive things that occurred in very early life can also actualize themselves, for example when a particular perfume is smelled again or the color of a person's eyes awakens an earlier feeling of happiness that one had connected with such eyes. Adalbert Stifter (1959) gives a good description of just such an early memory:

Way back in an empty nothingness there was something like bliss and delight, which grabbed me with force and penetrated into my being and almost destroyed me. It was not at all like anything in my present life. The characteristics which have stayed with me are: it was radiant and it was turbulent, it was below me. It must have been something very early because it seemed to me that it was surrounded by a huge, dark nothingness.

Then there was something else which came gently and with soothing into my heart. This characteristic was: it was sounds.

Then I was swimming in something that was gently wafting, I swam every now and again and everything became softer and softer until I felt as though I was drunk. Then there was nothing.

These three islands were lying, as in fairy tales and sagas, in the veiled ocean of the past, like the earliest folk memories.

The following climaxes became ever more distinct, the ringing of bells, a wide beam of light, a red sunset.

There was something which was very clear and which continuously repeated itself. A voice which spoke to me, eyes which looked at me and arms which soothed everything. I shouted for these things.

Then there was suffering, things unbearable and then sweetness and calming. I can remember striving and never reaching anything and then the cessation of terror and wretchedness. I can remember radiance and colour in my eyes and sounds in my ears and a feeling of sweetness in my whole being.

With increasing intensity, I felt the eyes that were looking at me, the voice which spoke to me, the arms which comforted me. I remember that I called it "Mom."

Once I felt these arms carrying me. They were dark spots on me. My memory told me later that they were forests outside of me. Then there was an experience like the first of my life, radiance and turbulence, then there was nothing. [p. 584]

EARLY MEMORIES IN DREAMS

Early memories can also express themselves in dreams, children's games, bodily sensations, unusual experiences, and exceptional situations. An example of a prenatal memory that actualized in a strange sleep-like state was reported by the American educationalist, Joseph Pearce (1978):

> I saw a large, red field looking as if it was made of glowing, red satin. . . . I was filled with respectful fear and astonishment. . . . I had the feeling that I had penetrated deep into

space. . . . I wanted to stay there forever. I felt the effects of
this experience for weeks afterwards, a warm feeling of
communion and power mixed with a strange longing, a sort
of homesickness. [p. 233]

We owe much to Frederick Kruse (1969), a psychotherapist from Wiesbaden, who over a period of many years made
a collection of such early memories as the above, from the
time of birth and before. Here are a few examples:

A 30-year-old woman, who had a very difficult birth, reported
an overwhelming experience which occurred as she was
taking a bath: "I almost suffocated in the warm water and in
my fear shouted for my husband. I had the feeling that
someone was strangling me. For ten minutes it was absolutely
terrible and then it slowly subsided. For several days after I
was terribly sensitive to noise and light." [p. 74]

Here is the example of an 8-year-old retarded boy who
seems to have managed to return to the damp security of his
mother's womb in the following way: "When one went into
his room in the morning, one did not at first notice anything
at all. He had crawled completely under the blankets. He lay
in this cave, completely soaked through with urine, clearly
contented. When asked what he was doing, he answered: 'I
am making steam for myself'" (p. 100).

Birth memories can also be hidden in everyday worries.
A 10-year-old child who had been born after a long and
difficult labor thought that he was going to suffocate every
time a piece of clothing, especially tight pullovers, was pulled
over his head.

Prenatal memories can be found very often in dreams.
A 30-year-old man who had been born with the umbilical

cord around his neck dreamt the following: "I fled to a cellar, the various exits were blocked, they found me there and put a noose around my neck. At the very last minute . . . a couple of people came to help me" (p. 125).

A 55-year-old woman reported having this dream:

> "I was sitting in a cave which is very narrow. The walls were hung with wet clothes. When I moved, the clothes gave way. Suddenly there was an earthquake. I was pressed with incredible force against a crack in the rocks near the exit of the cave. I had a terrible fear that I would not be able to get through and the feeling that I was suffocating. Somehow I was then pressed through. Outside I had to go through a waterfall. There was a harsh light and it was very cold." [p. 115]

Such dreams as these, like all other early memories, are put together using elements taken from various other experiences. In comparing the dream with the real event, one must decide in each individual case which elements of the dream actually lead us back to early events. The cases in which the dream contains elements of a real event that the dreamer did not previously know about, or where it was actually impossible for him to have known about it, are especially convincing. Many examples of just this phenomenon have now been documented and several will be discussed in Chapter 5, which is concerned with the reactivation of early experiences in the context of therapy.

Here is a final example of a birth trauma from a 45-year-old patient:

> "I was swimming under water, it was dark and very nice. All of a sudden I noticed that I urgently needed air. I could not get to the surface, however, because something was stopping me.

I tried frantically to go on. With utmost exertion, I eventually got to the top as if through a hole in the water. However, I still did not get any air because something was stuck around my head. Eventually someone forcibly tore the thing off me and at last I was able to breathe. There was bright sunshine. As I woke up, I gasped as if I really had been diving." [Kruse 1969, p. 143]

Several weeks later the patient found out that he had been a precipitate delivery and had been complete wrapped in the amnion. The first thing that the midwife did with considerable force and urgency was to free the newborn baby from the amnion, which was still stuck around his head. Only then had he been able to take his first breath.

FRAGMENTARY MEMORIES

Fragmentary memories of early experiences can also sometimes form connections with the person's ego, which developed later with the help of language. These fragments can then also be communicated in words. This has been especially observed in small children. Quite spontaneously or after they have been questioned about events in their infancy or during their birth, they can talk about what happened. The hypnotherapist David Chamberlain (1990) has collected examples of this. A friend from Santiago de Chile told the following story about his daughter:

"When she was 2 years old, he asked her if she could remember what it was like before she was born. She answered, 'It was so,' and put herself into exactly the same posture which the man could remember from an X-ray picture which had been made just before she had been born. The X-ray picture had been made because the labour was not normal and the unborn baby was in a poor condition. The picture revealed that she was in a breech position, her backside engaged in the pelvis instead of her head." [p. 150]

The body-memory had registered the situation before birth in exact detail and it was thus readily available for the child to recall.

A memory of the umbilical cord appears to be reflected in the following statement of a small girl:

"There was a snake in there with me . . . which tried to eat me but it wasn't a poisonous snake." She also talked about a dog that was there as well. She reported [that] it played with her so (she made rowing movements with her arms) and she had heard it barking. This improbable story about the dog was based upon the real little dog which the family procured as a pet about five months before the baby was born. The mother said that the dog had laid itself very often on her belly during the last months of the pregnancy. [p. 150]

Chamberlain also reports the story of a 2½-year-old girl who was born with the help of forceps. "Her mother asked her if was painful to be born. She answered: 'Yes, . . . like headache'" (p. 153).

UNDERSTANDING EARLY CHILDHOOD AMNESIA

These examples make it clear that the phenomenon of early childhood amnesia, that is, of the seeming loss of childhood memories, must be correctly understood. When the various ways in which early memories can express themselves are taken into consideration, then the problem appears in a different light. The appearance of prenatal experiences in children's painting, for example, has up until now received little attention. An art teacher, Wolfgang Grözinger (1984), reckons that it is possible to recognize several prenatal experiences in the small child's doodles. The feeling of rotating and floating in space can be seen, for example, in the rhythm of zig-zag lines or serial forms. Many children's drawings seem to represent the feeling of being in the uterus by cavelike circles, the umbilical cord and placenta symbolized by other elements in the picture. Terence Dowling, a prenatal therapist, has elucidated such connections in a comprehensive way using the pictures collected by Michaela Strauss, a German child psychotherapist (Strauss 1983, personal communications).

Apart from all this, there is a rapidly growing number of people who have gained emotional access to experiences that occurred in their infancy and at the time of their birth. The various techniques used to achieve this will be discussed in a later chapter. Not dissimilar from the people who in the first half of this century discovered the child within, many people have recently begun to discover not only the infant but also the unborn and newborn baby in themselves.

As soon as one talks about early memories, the question arises of whether such memories are only adult projections. Have adults only imagined the time before, during, or after their birth to be as they describe it? This question has to be raised anew and clarified in every individual case. However, a correct appreciation of how "real" early experiences are depends on a correct knowledge and understanding of the psychological abilities of the unborn and newborn child. The next chapter is dedicated to this issue. The abilities of the newborn child will be discussed first as these are better understood.

4

What Does the Unborn and Newborn Baby Feel? The Developmental Psychology of Early Childhood: Empirical Research

EVERY SMILE HAS MEANING

In the last few years, a great change has taken place in the way in which science looks at babies. Before this, most scientists were only able to see a primitive bundle of reflexes in the small child. Now science is rediscovering what observant parents have always known. So, for example, scientists have now confirmed that the infant is an active, little person, with feelings and perceptions, who relates intensively to his environment and is greatly influenced by it. Quite surprised, scientists observe how even the newborn child follows objects and people with his eyes, exhibits quite clear perceptual preferences, can recognize patterns, and prefers what he already knows (Field 1982). There was great amazement when it was first observed that, for example, even the smallest baby can mimic adults (Meltzoff and Moore 1977). The newborn baby's hearing has also now been proved to be completely developed. The small baby follows voices that he knows and can distinguish complex sounds from one another. Even the ability of the fetus to experience "olfactory" learning is experimentally proved (Hepper 1995).

The experience that many parents know well, that babies can be deeply moved when one talks to them, has now been objectively confirmed by research using film. This shows that the baby follows the rhythm and melody of the voice and, for example, moves with the voice of its mother and answers her with a sort of dance (Condon and Sander 1974). These movements in response to being spoken to have now also been filmed in utero. Numerous studies have also demonstrated that the other senses, for example taste and touch, and balance are all developed and function in a sophisticated way by the time of birth. Curiously enough, it was only the objectification through the use of film and serial photography that first allowed scientists to really notice the enormous amount of information that streams back and forth in the mother–child relationship (Papousek 1979). No one seriously doubts any longer that this remarkable activity, these perceptual abilities and the intensity of interaction are experienced by the child. However, limiting remarks are still frequently found in the literature and derogatory adjectives, such as *primitive, rudimentary,* and *reflex-like* are still often applied. Nevertheless, a shift in attitude can be observed and this in turn is leading to further and more interesting research. It is generally true that each improvement in the method of research leads to a higher evaluation of the psychological abilities of the baby.

The more sophisticated the test, the easier it is to see just how competent even the smallest baby is.

Psychologists have always managed to invent ever more complex conditioning experiments. Here is an example that David Chamberlain (1990) reported:

> Experimenters built on the fact that infants usually turn their heads to the side where they are touched on the cheek. Normally, they will do this about 30 percent of the time. By making a sweet solution available when the baby turned its head, the rate was raised to 83 percent. Once established at that level, infants were taught to turn their heads to the left at the sound of a bell and right at the sound of a buzzer to obtain the sugar solution. Infants quickly learned the sweet taste of success.
>
> The signals were then reversed and the reward given for turns in the opposite direction. Infants who had learned bell-left and buzzer-right now had to forget this and learn bell-right and buzzer-left in order to get the reward. A gradual shift in behavior took place, producing a reliable effect once again. Newborns mastered all these moves in thirty minutes. [p. 43]

This experiment also showed that babies with difficult births learn more slowly. Furthermore, various studies have shown the importance of emotional contact after birth. The duration of the emotional contact immediately after birth influences the closeness and intensity of the mother–child relationship many months later. Babies who are allowed to remain with their mothers after birth smiled more and cried less than babies who had experienced separation. Babies who were more often carried in their mother's arms had an increased weight gain and quicker growth rate than babies who were left in their cradles (Klaus and Kennell 1983).

The intensity of the very earliest learning processes is made very apparent in studies that demonstrate how prenatal experiences remain active. In one experiment, newborn babies could choose which voice they heard over a loudspeaker by varying the intensity of their sucking on a dummy or pacifier. They showed clear preference for their mother's voice and the sound of her heartbeat to the voice of their father (DeCasper and Fifer 1980, Kolata 1984).

Just how important is it to respect newborn babies and their many abilities and to treat them in a caring way immediately after their birth is shown in the following observation: In hospitals and clinics where care is taken to ensure that newborn babies have a "gentle landing," the usual and allegedly "physiological weight loss" after birth does not occur. It only happens when the babies are treated roughly and in an unfriendly way. This is particularly true for premature and low-weight babies. Ruth Rice (1986) has demonstrated that when these babies are caressed and experience body contact and massage, they grow more quickly and their development catches up sooner.

A typical example of the general attitude of scientists to babies can be seen in the fact that in less recent textbooks true smiling was only accredited to them at the end of their first year of life! This particular age has always had a downward tendency. Now it is recognized that babies clearly demonstrate "social smiling" when they are just 6 weeks old. One can only agree with David Chamberlain (1990) when he states that it is long overdue that we accept "that every baby smile has a meaning" (p. 60). Because even premature babies smile, we can be more or less certain that the fetus also smiles. Just how sensitive babies are to mimicry was shown in an experiment in which mothers were told to look unhappy in the presence of their babies. The babies began to cry almost immediately, looked away from their mothers and even days later reacted with a certain mistrust (Tronick and Adamson 1980).

RELATING IN THE WOMB

Until a few years ago, it was only possible to feel the unborn child and it was only noticed when it moved. Nowadays with the help of modern technology—intrauterine photography and ultrasound—it has become possible to see the baby. The first photo of the little newcomer is the ultrasound picture. This has added a new dimension to the relationship of the parents to their unborn child. The relationship is more direct and the child somehow more real. The effect is similar to that caused by the film studies of infants that objectified the mother–child relationship. For adults, visibility seems to make things more real. Thus, I now quote some of the descriptions of the behavior of the fetus in its uterine world that the psychoanalyst, Alessandra Piontelli (1987) reported from her longitudinal study of fetal development using ultrasound:

> During the ultrasound investigation, Julia seemed to be extremely calm but not immobile. Most of the time, she drifted around in the amniotic water in time to her mother's breathing as if she was being cradled. More than once it was observed how she rocked herself rhythmically, apparently in order to go to sleep. Most of the time she held her arm by her side but sometimes also between her legs or she brought her hands together and moved her fingers with great dexterity. However, most remarkable of all were the permanent movements of her tongue. Julia seemed to be permanently busy

with it, playing with it by sticking it out between her lips and then pulling it back in. In the last observation, we saw her passionately licking the placenta. . . . Once she also licked the umbilical cord. As I watched her, Julia gave me the impression that she had a peaceful temperament, living in harmony with her intrauterine world. [p. 457]

Little James behaved as follows in the womb:

He hardly moved and lay crouched up in a corner of the womb, covering his eyes and face with his hands and arms. It almost looked as though he was also using his legs to protect his face. His immobility did not give the impression of calm as did Julia's drifting around. It seemed to stem from tension. He was not exactly in panic but he was definitely not calm. With his arms around his head, his eyes and face covered, he looked like one of the figures which Munch painted. . . . Even the tight space of the womb seemed to be too big for him. It was almost impossible to see his face . . . frequently we saw the umbilical cord between his arms and legs but it was impossible to say whether he was doing something with it or whether he was just holding it. . . . The only thing that was easy to observe was the occasional erection. [p. 460]

And now a passage from the description of twins:

The girl seemed to be livelier than the boy, even though she was smaller. She moved her hands and arms, her head and feet frequently. She rubbed her feet, yawned, bent her legs, stretched her neck, stretched her legs, folded her hands and took her finger in her mouth. . . . She seemed to be alive and interested in trying out various movements, positions and sensations. She looked like somebody who is interested in what is around them and in their own life. . . . Her brother gave a completely different impression although he also moved more often. He appeared disquiet as though he was permanently searching for a perfect peace. . . . As an assistant remarked, he used the placenta as a cushion. . . . I had the impression that every stimulus bothered him. . . . He answered every nudge from his sister by turning away and even buried his face deeper into a remote corner of his placenta. When she did not give up in her attempts to contact him and continued to touch him quite carefully with her hands and feet, he reacted by pushing her away fiercely. She immediately looked shocked by his strength. [pp. 413–426]

The continuity between the prenatal and postnatal patterns of behavior was particularly apparent to Piontelli. The ways in which the children behaved in the womb and then outside of it even years later when they were small children were almost identical. A connection with the mother's behavior was difficult to establish. Perhaps there was a connection in the case of little James, who sat so fearful in the corner of the uterus. His mother was plagued by terrible fear. The surprising difference in the ways the twins arranged themselves in their respective parts of the womb was most remarkable. A definite conclusion to be drawn from Piontelli's work is that basic mannerisms and orientations in the individual child's behavior begin to develop in its relationship to its twin during their uterine life together.

If one wants to gain a correct appreciation of life before birth, it is important to remember that the unborn child experiences and perceives—even when we can only infer that by observing its external behavior. It is often possible to see fetal experience quite undisguised in psychotic patients. For this reason, the report of the Swiss psychoanalyst and psychiatrist Gaetano Benedetti (1983a), about a psychotic patient will be quoted here in connection with the above-mentioned observations about twins. This patient had been born with a twin sister who had been dead for a long time and was mummified—a "fetus papyraceus" as gynecologists call it. It was probable that the twin had died in the middle of the pregnancy as a result of a bad allergic shock that the mother had experienced. However, this was not known at the time when the patient, the surviving twin, became ill:

> During her puberty, the patient had experienced the follow-ing fantasy several times: If she had had a twin brother, she would have been happier. She would have experienced him almost as a part of her own self instead of being in competi-tion with a brother. During this same period, the patient had had an oft-recurring dream. She saw a parrot which was trapped in a cage and which had sexual intercourse through the bars with a dead bird which was fastened onto the cage outside. Both birds seemed to be floating in a particular room. Another dream was about an unmarried woman who had separated herself from her friend. A second woman, who was symbiotically attached to the first woman, carried the "physical remains" of the male person who had disappeared in a plastic sack. She often spoke with the disintegrated male body which was contained there. A peculiar symbiotic fantasy.
> [Benedetti 1983a, unpublished lecture]

In the seventh week of prenatal development, motor abilities are such that there are general movements of avoidance and attention; in the sixteenth week, mimicry; seventeenth week, regular breathing movements; twenty-fourth week, the ability to cry; from the middle of the pregnancy, the ability to make complex movements. With regard to perception, the first sense to mature is that of the skin perceptions in about the seventh week. The sense of balance is completely developed by about the sixteenth week, and hearing by about the twenty-fifth week. At about the same time, the senses of taste and sight and the registration of pressure, pain, and cold have all developed. The unborn child reacts strongly to music, shows a preference for Mozart and Vivaldi, and can defend itself very forcibly against rock music. It reacts to loud noises with an increase in heart rate. The same response occurs when the mother gets excited. In particular, the mother's stress hormones cross the placenta and affect the baby (see Bürgin 1982, Chamberlain 1983).

The unborn child is just like the newborn in that it is permanently learning and coming to terms with everything new in its environment. The learning processes seem to be incredibly intensive. The child registers even the most subtle changes. For example, not only can it distinguish directly after its birth its mother's voice from that of its father and recognize songs that it heard in the womb, but it can also distinguish between nursery rhymes read to it during the pregnancy from those it has never heard before. One woman had learned to play the flute while she was pregnant, and she observed that after the birth playing the flute always calmed the baby. But the effect only occurred when the mother played the flute. The baby remained unmoved when it heard music played by the much better sounding flute virtuoso, Frans Brueggen.

All that is learned in the womb remains extremely influential in later life. This is most likely the reason why the sound of the mother's heartbeat has such a calming effect after birth. Infants who have been separated from their mothers but who are played the sound of the mother's heartbeat from a cassette show a much better weight increase than the babies in a control group (Salk 1973). The calming effect of the maternal heartbeat, concludes Salk, has led mothers quite unconsciously to carry their child almost always on their left arm. This is, according to Salk, the reason that in 80 percent of all paintings of Mary and the baby Jesus, she is holding Jesus to her left side.

Prenatal learning processes begin very early. Even the ability of premature babies, born in the fifth month of pregnancy, to recognize voices is influenced by the frequency characteristics of its own mother's voice (Truby et al. 1965). Prenatal hearing has a measurable effect on later language ability. When a child in the womb hears and learns about music, this experience has a positive effect on its later musical ability. Experience in prenatal learning programs points in the same direction.

THE BABY'S FEELINGS DURING BIRTH

With this background on the behavior, perceptions, and learning abilities of the fetus, we can more easily trust our spontaneous impression and once and for all dismiss the idea that the child does not experience anything of its own birth. Newborn babies are just all too often the picture of misery. In the eighteenth century, Erasmus Darwin (1731–1802), Charles Darwin's grandfather, demonstrating an empathy way ahead of his time, wrote the following:

> The first and strongest sensations which forced themselves upon the boy after his birth were caused by shortness of breath and constriction of his chest and then the sudden transition from a temperature of over 37 degrees to our cold climate. The child shivered, that means, he moved all his muscles one after the other in order to free himself from the pressure on his chest and he began to draw air in short, quick

breaths. At the same time, the cold penetrated his flushed skin so that it slowly turned pale. His bladder and bowels emptied out their contents and this first experience of something awful led to fear which itself is nothing other than the expectation of a horrible experience. This premature combination of movements and feelings remains so for the whole of later life. Fear makes the skin turn cold and pale and produces shivering, acceleration of breathing and the emptying of bladder and bowels. As a result, these manifestations have become the natural and universal expressions of this emotion. [quoted in Jones 1923, p. 120]

Over one hundred years later, Freud (1972) described the effects of the fear we experience during birth in a similar way. And the midwife, Dorothy Garley (1924), published an article entitled "The Shock of Being Born," in which she collects her observations:

In such cases [narrow pelvis], there is no doubt that terrible fear occurs as a result of the asphyxia produced by the greatly diminished circulation. Under these circumstances either children are born dead or it is only possible to resuscitate them with great difficulty. That the children are aware of the impending suffocation can be seen in the fact that in the period between contractions they wriggle around in the uterus. They look exactly like the movements which every creature makes when it is drowning. When one sees such desperate movements during a birth, there is little chance of the child being born alive. Even when the child's body successfully withstands the danger, then the after-effects of the fear and feeling of suffocation remain quite apparent. [p. 136]

Garley gives a graphic description of the uncertainty the child must come to terms with after its birth:

The child must get used to the feeling of uncertainty which is
caused by the lack of what was before always there, always
tangible, the protective wall of the uterus. Now when the
child reaches out, it feels nothing, its leg moves freely into
empty space. The feeling of security is replaced by the feeling
of insecure isolation. The child must get used to being
touched by hands where before it was only cradled. [p. 155]

Garley was prepared even those many years ago to
specify the traumatic aspects of a difficult birth:

Now when the pressure which results from every contraction
causes the mother such terrible pain, why should the child
not experience exactly the same? These pains then would be
the very first feelings which the child experiences and they
have such a marked effect on the child because the contrast
to the pleasure it previously enjoyed is so extreme. . . .
Because there is normally a certain disproportion between
the size of the baby's head and the exit through the pelvis,
then there is always squeezing, pressing and moulding of the
head until it has conformed to the pelvic opening and can
pass through. Each of the contractions, which occur with
intervals of from three to five minutes and sometimes more
frequently, helps a little. However, many strong contractions,
which often must be endured for days and nights, are
necessary when the pelvis is narrow and the head very big.
Even when the head has survived this stage and has reached
the vaginal canal and begun to go through, the exit still has
to be forcibly enlarged by the head as it comes down. As a
result of this, the head is sometimes pressed so thin and the
brain inside it so squeezed, that the bones slide together, the
space between them disappearing, one then lying over the
other, the posterior cranial bone disappears completely under the parietal bone and the middle of the stern protrudes
in a sharp edge. This overlapping of the bones disappears

again at the latest 48 hours after the birth but the head retains a form which is a lifelong souvenir of its forcible displacement. Is it feasible to presume that such pressure can occur without producing pain or without having a deep and lasting effect upon the psychological life of the newborn child? [p. 145]

With much psychological insight, the experienced midwife gives a vivid description of the three phases of birth—the phase of opening, of descent, and then of expulsion:

In the first phase, the child's head is pressed between two rings. One is the neck of uterus muscle which gradually expands so that sooner or later every place on the head is put under pressure. The other is the hard ring of bone which forms the exit through the pelvis in which . . . the pressure also gradually proceeds as the head is moulded. . . . His whole body is pressed together into a solid mass by the walls of muscle and is then used as a ram to force the head down and to pound it through the bony ring. All this can take hours!

Nature has provided an interesting way for the maternal ring of bone to be able to enlarge. A cartilage in the middle allows the ring to dilate. However, an enormous amount of strength is needed to achieve even just a little movement. . . . During very difficult forceps deliveries, it cannot be avoided that the head is so squeezed that deep pressure marks are left on the cheeks and around the ears. . . . It should not be forgotten that during a forceps delivery the doctor must often pull on the child's head using his whole strength. When such a child is later touched by someone, it connects this touch with the idea of an increase in pain and begins to cry. . . . To a certain extent what has just been mentioned might explain why some children from the very

beginning shy away from human touch or at least are
frightened of it for a long time.

The second phase of the process of birth begins when
the head has had enough moulding and pressing and has
withstood the difficulty of getting through the pelvis. It is
then forced to enter the vaginal canal. Here it is confronted
by new discomforts. The main pressure extends now to
another sensitive area: the face, the eyes and eye-sockets and
the nose. . . . Can one presume that such strong pressure
on such a well-innervated surface does not cause pain and
does not leave behind it the impression of a painful experience in the psyche? Is it possible that this further pressure
marks a serious intensification of the pain suffered in the first
phase? The contractions press the fetus into a solid mass and
then there is the problem of what to do with the hands and
knees. The face is bent down towards the chest, the strongest
pressure being exerted by the cone of the uterus against the
back of the head. The knees are thus forced up against the
face. In this position one can conclude that it is highly
probable that the eye-balls must withstand very strong pressure from the hands or the knees.

Because the child experiences pain when the eye-balls
are pressed directly after birth—it cries immediately when
they are touched—one must presume that it is capable of
experiencing the same thing before its birth. . . . The nose
is pressed flat against the mother's coccyx and is thereby
sometimes injured. The eye-sockets are squashed against the
strong vaginal muscles when it becomes necessary for them to
expand in order to let the head through. When it is the
woman's first birth, this dilation phase lasts many hours
during which the pressure on the face remains undiminished.
As soon as the head is through, one must grasp for the
umbilical cord which is often wrapped tightly around the
child's neck as many as three times. Usually it takes only a
matter of seconds to pull the loops over the head but one

must not forget that the feeling of suffocation during the birth is increased by the tightness of the cord and this is not only because of the partial interruption of the circulation in the umbilical cord but also because of the obstruction of the circulation in the throat. Many children cannot tolerate the slightest feeling of something tight around their throat. They scream and pull on every scarf long before they can feel it as tight. However, even the hint of tightness caused by a scarf can awaken the chain of memories which leads back to this first experience connected with birth. . . . Being washed is normally a shock for the child. Because one is never sure exactly when the baby will be born, the water used to disinfect the eyes has usually cooled. In any case, the child coughs because of the temperature contrast and cries. However, when the crying is not loud enough for the nurse, then she grabs the child by the heels, swings it up-side-down through the air and hits it hard between the shoulders. As a result the whole body bends suddenly backwards, the child takes a deep breath and begins to cry loudly. The crying is not only with dilated lungs but with all the signs of great distress and helplessness. It has exactly the same sound as when an older child has received an angry slap or been painfully disappointed because something has been forbidden him. It must be a bitter experience to come out of the cosy world of the womb into a sudden bath of cold air and head hanging down to be greeted with a hefty smack.—Truly it would be hard treatment for an adult who had been toughened by discomfort but a shocking experience for a sensitive, newborn child. This may explain why otherwise good lads and men show a disproportionate sensitivity when, in harmless friendship, they are unexpectedly thumped between the shoulders. Some nurses hit so hard and violently as though the weak bundle were a naughty child which needs strict punishment and not gentle encouragement. The dreadful crying, with quivering lower lip and contorted face makes one feel that one should not hit. . . .

Now when the child is crying satisfactorily, it is confronted by the next horror. It is laid flat on the bed where it rolls around helplessly. This experience can be seen as a real shock because up until then every movement, every push had touched something. Warm, protective walls were all-embracing. Now there is only empty space and cold air, absolute vulnerability—, and for the first time there is the painful experience of being completely alone—there is nothing at hand which reflects the familiar feeling of physical togetherness and psychological security. Even his own crying is to the child a terrible, unfamiliar and unknown noise. The flat surface of the bed and the position of the back increase still further the feeling of insecurity. . . . Finally, the child is crying in complete panic and is shaking in all his members. . . . It sometimes takes a long time until children have come to terms with the fear of lying on their backs. One may ask here whether this early remembering of fear and helplessness in a prostrate position can have a certain influence on female sexuality.

Also the effect of light on the psyche seems to be of great significance. It is, for example, interesting to learn that a neurotic person's fear of light can be connected with the authority of the father. It is certain that a child born under present circumstances [i.e., the beginning of the 1920s, author's note] in a hospital or maternity clinic or apartment with electric light suffers from the excess of bright light which falls for the first time in his life directly into his sensitive eye-balls when he is lying on his back under a lamp. Because the visual nerve is so suddenly subjected to light to which it is not accustomed, pain occurs which also has psychological consequences. Whoever doubts this must only lie for ten minutes with his face looking up into a bright light which—as is usual in hospitals and clinics—has a white lamp-shade which intensifies the light. Add to that white walls and ceilings, the white aprons of the nurses and the white linen on the beds. Even eyes which are used to light feel great discomfort. Ten minutes go by before the child is brought into another position. During this time, it is crying most probably quite pitifully because of all the hardship it must bear after its birth. One can observe how it often stops crying and tries to open its eyes naturally but the pain caused by the bright light is so strong that it breaks again into tears, as it were in protest against the cause of pain. [pp. 146ff]

I have quoted this English midwife so extensively because I hold her article, which appeared in the *Internationale Zeitschrift für Psychoanalyse* in 1924, to be a testimony of human empathy and courageous truthfulness. One finds a large number of suggestions in the article that have already been incorporated into modern, obstetrical practice. Dorothy Garley's writing broke through the taboo against speaking honestly and openly about the danger of birth and of being born. We know that only a few psychoanalysts had the strength and determination to be open on this point. One of them is Phyllis Greenacre (1945), who in the 1940s wrote articles about the biographical significance of the birth trauma. She remarked, with a certain intuition, "But perhaps birth is unavoidably and narrowly connected in our feelings with death. Perhaps the struggle to be born is so terrible and so overwhelming for us that it is not possible for us to consider it with scientific neutrality. Perhaps men have too much fear of expulsion and women too much direct fear" (p. 51).

Ever since the end of the last century, courageous obstetricians have time and again made public how even apparently normal births are connected with internal injuries, especially inside the skull. As early as 1924, Hans Saenger, along with Philip Schwartz, one of the pioneers in this research, wrote succinctly: "During the birth of present day, civilised human beings, such an enormous force acts upon the child's brain that birth must be classified as a trauma, the extent and danger of which can only be imagined by someone who has quite frequently had the opportunity to dissect the skulls of newborn children" (p. 17). This fundamental statement can nowadays be supported by increasingly convincing evidence.

Of course there are births that proceed in a completely different way. It well may be that some children arrive fully awake and with a lively curiosity. They are undoubtedly in a highly alert state that one can understand as stemming from the "Eustress" of the birth. In the period after birth, babies seem to be receptive in a quite special way for impressions and relationships. One can guess that bonds are made at this time that can encourage a deep, lifelong confidence in human relationships. The analysis of films has proven that when mother and child are not separated after the birth but can remain together, they communicate much more intensely with one another in the months thereafter (Klaus and Kennel 1983).

It may well be that positive feelings of victory and triumph and of liberation can stem from this first experience of a successful birth. The applause of a jubilant crowd may be just so intense because it connects internally with the joy and exaltation that people who are privileged to be present at the arrival of another human being can experience.

Despite all of this, I believe that, especially in the recent past, we have used the positive aspects of birth to deny the dangers involved and to repress the agonies of birth by unrealistic idealization. Much supports the notion that, because of the antagonistic forces that were active during evolution, human birth has as a rule a traumatic aspect or at least always involves being stressed to the limits (Müller 1991). Thus there is a necessity to use all resources and forces possible to deal with this problem. It seems to me that this presupposes that we face up to the depths of despair and terrors of birth and their significance for the historical development of human experience. Under so-called natural conditions, perinatal mortality and birth stress, at least in the high cultures, were always extremely high.

This subject matter is, however, so complex that it must be approached in the following sections of the book from several different directions. Nevertheless we are already in a position to conclude that, for the sensitive and responsive child about to be born, the stressful experience of birth has very often the character of nothing less than a terrible shock, a catastrophe and even an annihilation. All too often, babies after birth look as though they have been mishandled. The presumption mentioned at the beginning of this chapter that the child is not aware of what happens to it is in my opinion only evidence of our massive denial. On the other hand, it is known that the concentration of opioid substances, so-called antistress hormones, in the umbilical cord and in the amniotic fluid during birth is much increased and that this signifies that there is a certain protection against stress (Genazzini 1989, Lou 1989). It also explains the altered state of attention that the newborn baby presents. In good circumstances birth can be something like an ecstatic adventure and peak experience. Because of their significance, the traumatic aspects of birth will now be drawn together in a single exposition.

THE TRAUMATIC ASPECTS OF BIRTH

Our understanding of the psychosomatic processes involved in birth is still in its infancy. Only a few of the facts that would lead to a fuller understanding have as yet been discerned. It is easy to forget that the Dick-Read and Lamaze methods of supporting a woman during labor, both of which are nowadays so familiar, were developed only in the 1940s. The gentle birth movement encouraged by Frederick Leboyer, which pays particular attention to the needs of the child during birth, appeared only during the 1970s. A comprehensive understanding of the process of birth, including an understanding of the complex psychosocial factors that influence how a birth progresses, is only being developed at the present time.

As has already been mentioned, up until the nineteenth century the process of birth was embedded in the realm of ritual, traditional practices, and superstition (Gélis 1989, Kuntner 1986). From the nineteenth century until the present day, birth has been medicalized in a comprehensive way. What is now called perinatal medicine includes care of the newborn and has led to a dramatic reduction in perinatal mortality—at the moment less than 0.1 percent. However, this development has a dark side. Mother and child have been progressively estranged. The psychological dimension has been lost from view and the instinctive energies and fundamental needs of both mother and child during the birth process have been disregarded. The development of prenatal psychology and the concern that birth should be as natural as possible are expressions of a desire to understand birth anew as an event of fundamental human significance. As a result of women's new self-understanding, an ever-increasing volume of literature has appeared with many reports of birth from the point of view of the mother. However, in the desire for gentle birth, the situation of her child during the birth has not been neglected.

One reason for this development is that human birth is an event that pushes us to the utmost limits and at the same time forms the foundation for our feelings toward ourselves and toward life. Human birth, because of evolutionary, biological reasons, is a trauma. Nevertheless, hidden within it is the possibility of an ecstatic and transformative experience for both mother and child. To approach the question of the psychological trauma involved in birth—and thereby also the question of the therapy for such primal wounds—I now present the aspects of birth that are traumatic at the somatic and physiological level. Actually we can only infer the psychological wounds that birth can give rise to when we produce a synthesis using information collected from observation of the somatic, the physiological, and the behavioral levels, with inferences drawn from the reliving of birth fear in therapeutic situations. First we look at the somatic level, the damage done to the brain by birth.

As early as the nineteenth century, brain hemorrhage was diagnosed as the cause of death of the newborn in many cases. A more systematic study, however, was begun only in the 1920s and is connected especially with the name of Philip Schwartz. He was able to show that birth damage to the newborn and also to children who in other respects seemed to be healthy occurred far more frequently than had been previously supposed. This fact showed itself in the multifarious illnesses that ensued. The damage to the child after birth is often so obvious and leads to mental deficiency, convulsions, and paralysis. But it is important in connection with our concerns here to realize that minimal damage occurs much more often than earlier presumed. Schwartz (1968) writes:

> Lamed, crippled, mentally deficient and epileptic victims of the processes of birth are certainly a heavy burden to bear for a society which feels itself responsible for these unfortunate creatures. However, there is also a numerically much larger group of damaged people whose defects can only be proved by especially careful investigation. Many of these find a place in society although they will probably never be able to attain their genetically determined level of productivity. The relevant investigations have proven that damage to the brain during birth is of the greatest aetiological significance for conditions in childhood which are described as psychopathy, neurosis, educational deficiency, disturbances of behaviour and defects of character. And often enough there seems to be a connection with tendency towards crime. [p. 2390]

Schwartz understood the damage to be caused above all by compression of the brain as well as lack of oxygen and the "atmospheric suction" that is activated after the membrane rupture by the internal pressure in the uterus during the contractions. This is the most important force leading to the delivery of the fetus from the uterus and which thereby assaults the part of the body that is most prominent, most usually the head. This often overwhelming minor pressure during the process of birth produces the birth swelling and can not only reverse the flow of blood in the large cerebral blood vessels but even bring it to a complete standstill. "Compression of the skull and the inferior pressure after the delivery shatter the substance of the brain. . . . No wonder that the newborn enters the world very often in a state of shock, is or appears to be half dead. If it could speak, how often would we hear: 'It was horrific! It would have been better to remain unborn!'" (p. 2386).

Recently, the gynecologist Hermann Kurrek (1986) has described the traumatic aspects of birth more precisely:

The increasing pressure of the contractions of ten or more kilograms results not only in disturbance of the cerebral circulation (blood flow in the brain) and irreversible tissue displacement accompanied by parenchymnecrosis (death of brain tissue) and haemorrhage (formation of blood clots). From the configuration of the skull and face bones, indentation of the Formanen occipitale magnum (the hole at the base of the skull leading to the vertebral column) appears with the danger of penetrating the Medulla oblongata (the brain stem). During a woman's first delivery, this compression of the brain extends over a period of between 15 to 24 hours. In following deliveries, it lasts between 10 and 12 hours. From the first contraction onwards there is a recurring danger of hypoxia (lack of oxygen) lasting between 20 and 60 seconds and during the final contractions of between 1 and 2 minutes. [p. 305]

It is Kurrek's opinion that every birth leads to much bruising of the brain. The results of the investigations carried out by the Russian child neurologist, Alexander Ratner (1991), are significant in this connection. In a serial study of schoolchildren, he found that about 75 percent showed minor neurological deficiencies that he understood as a result of birth trauma.

If one reads the careful study by the neuropediatrician Dagobert Müller (1973), entitled *Displacement of the Brain during Birth,* Kurrek's statements do not seem improbable. It is significant that, after many years of research, Müller himself is convinced that evolution has led to human birth pathology and that this in turn means that every birth has a traumatic aspect. In the book, which appeared in 1973, he was unwilling to draw this conclusion because his opinion at that time was that birth as a "natural event" cannot involve any pathology. In a letter to me, he writes:

> In the first version of the book, we still believed in a certain evolutionary teleology—in the sense that everything is "normal" and had therefore formulated that "nature" would not have built a process necessary for the preservation of a species upon a pathology. Only through consideration of comparative obstetrics . . . did it become clear that with the evolution of mankind a primary pathology—one can even call it an evolutionary pathology—occurred. As a result I must confess today that human birth is normally traumatic. Whether this trauma always becomes a pathology is another question. In any case, the birth trauma is a further influence upon the genetic individuality in ways that can be analysed in each case. [1989, personal communication]

In the next few years, we will be able to get a much clearer picture of what actually happens at birth using modern investigative processes. Computed tomography has already shown that hidden hemorrhages caused by birth are far more frequent than was assumed and also than previously could be proven (Ludwig 1983). It is to be expected that spin tomography will produce even more reliable data. Furthermore, research projects have been planned involving computer simulation by which our knowledge of the mechanics of birth should be greatly deepened. Even so, when the mechanics of birth are considered, a crucial statement about the traumatic aspects of human birth can already be made (Wischnik 1989). Put bluntly, a single centimeter is lacking. The diameter of the child's head and the diameter of the middle of the pelvis measure about 10 centimeters. At least 1 centimeter is missing for the soft parts. This centimeter is gained by deformation of the child's skull. That is the crux of the birth trauma from the somatic point of view. On the physiological level, the traumatic aspect of birth can be approached using the concept of *experimental neurosis* proposed by the Russian physiologist Ivan Pavlov (1849–1936) and the concept of "distress" expounded by the Austrian-Canadian doctor and biochemist Hans Selye (1974). According to Pavlov, an experimental neurosis is the result of overstimulation or the hopeless confusion caused by simultaneous positive and negative reinforcement. It is interesting and suggestive that Pavlov observed a case of "traumatic" reaction to a powerful "stimulus" when his laboratory was flooded. The test animals, in this case dogs, could only be rescued very near to drowning. According to his observation, this event had an effect like "the one which can be justly compared with traumatic neurosis in humans" (Pavlov 1955, p. 338). It is also to be noted that all the dogs had "forgotten" their conditioned reflex. Perhaps the same happens to us: what we have learned in the womb gets lost because of the traumatic elements of human birth.

Pavlov understood experimental neuroses as unregulated, persisting nervous activities. Clinically they are characterized, as has also been observed in humans, by marked behavioral disturbance and disorganization and all sorts of psychosomatic symptoms. What Pavlov described as experimental neurosis is equivalent to what is called in stress research exhaustion reaction. This is the response to continuous and irresolvable stress. Very similar disorganization of behavior and various psychosomatic symptoms can be observed. The English psychotherapist and perinatal psychologist Frank Lake (1979) made some very creative suggestions in this regard. The concepts of Pavlov and Selye can be fruitfully used to comprehend the traumatic aspects of birth on the physiological level. The traumatic aspect of birth would then work like transmarginal stress, producing the response of unbearable fear, panic, and pain, and eventually leading to the collapse of normal behavior. In this state, everything is turned against one's own body and the organism desires nothing other than to die and be destroyed. This corresponds on the physiological level to the paradoxical and ultraparadoxical reaction: weak stimuli lead them to strong responses; strong stimuli to weak responses; aversive, repulsive stimuli receive a positive answer; and positive stimuli trigger pain and defensiveness. What just before was avoided as painful, can now in a most peculiar way actually be desired. On the psychological level, we may presume with Lake that this condition corresponds to a state of absolute helplessness and terror. Death becomes the only hope. Which psychotherapist has not met patients who come to him in this state?

In psychoanalysis, the concept of experimental neurosis or exhaustion syndrome corresponds to the so-called actual neurosis, that is, a neurotic disorder due to overstimulation. This includes the traumatic neuroses, the neurasthenic reaction, and the anxiety neurosis (Janus 1987). It is clear from Freud's statements that he in fact implicitly described these three forms of neurosis as determined by birth trauma. At first, Freud guessed that the anxiety neurosis and the neurasthenic reaction had a sexual disorder as their autonomous cause. However, in later years he emphasized the connection with the birth trauma. He stated that with a sexual disturbance a direct fear can appear, "that is, a state is produced in which the self stands helpless before an enormous tension of desires which like birth itself ends in fear" (Freud 1963, p. 127). Insofar as every neurosis goes back to an actual neurotic core, according to psychoanalytic theory, then a relationship to birth trauma is immediately specified for neurotic and psychosomatic symptom formation (Janus 1989b). This connection was not completely realized in traditional psychoanalytic teachings and its further development. As a result the discovery of the significance of the psychotraumatic aspects of birth in primal and LSD therapy appears as a sort of rediscovery—at least if one ignores the sidestreams within psychoanalysis associated with the names of the Swiss psychoanalyst Graber and the Hungarian psychoanalyst Fodor.

Whereas the traumatic aspect of birth on the somatic-anatomical level is immediately to be seen in the bruising and deformation of the head, transmarginal stress is naturally a fleeting phenomenon. It is known that levels of stress hormone during birth increase markedly, and when there are complications they become extremely high. Equally, the changes in heart rate that can be measured during birth provide an indication of the levels of stress involved. The direct observation of the newborn child and the pediatric examination also allow a certain check to be made. However, the Apgar score, a point-system used to estimate the vital functions of the newborn, is unclear and not so reliable. This at least is my impression from discussions with various birth assistants. According to the figures given by Schwartz, about 30 percent of babies are "quite exhausted" after their birth. According to the rough estimates made by midwives and obstetricians whom I have asked, about a further 30 percent are "clearly exhausted." That would mean that about 30 to 70 percent of newborns have experienced a state of transmarginal stress. Such a figure is at the present time speculative. Research is required in this area, especially in reconciling results from different levels of observation. A favorable development in this direction is the contact that has been initiated between perinatal medicine and perinatal psychology (Janus 1993b, 1995, Klimek 1992).

There is a very detailed body of empirical evidence concerning the aftereffects of traumatic childhood experiences such as mishandling, sexual abuse, and accident (Horowitz 1976, Terr 1991). These childhood traumas later have impact on the person's experience and behavior, again and again, in the form, for example, of hallucinations, behavioral disorders, specific phobias, superstitious fears, perceptual disturbances, denial, semiconsciousness, and loss of temper. The flashbacks of the traumatic situation have their equivalent in the actualization of traumatic pre- and perinatal experiences in psychotherapy.

Whatever the relationship between stronger and milder stress during birth may be, much evidence indicates that birth has a traumatic effect on the psychology of the newborn as an experience of overwhelming fear of annihilation and general emotional shock. There is also much evidence that the ability of the child to come to terms with the traumatic aspects of its birth is determined by the way in which the child is received by its parents and introduced to the world. Statistical studies are completely unequivocal on this point. Birth trauma followed by family conflict and social strain burden a person's life and development in a most extreme way. This fact is confirmed daily in the treatment of individuals in psychotherapy.

The previous chapters and the presentation of more objective observations about the experience of birth and prenatal life are intended to facilitate correct evaluation of the information from psychotherapy that stems from subjective observation of personal experience. This information about the reliving of pre- and perinatal experiences forms a central part of this book. The plausibility of the case studies will depend on how successfully and how convincingly it can be demonstrated that experience from our time in the womb, from birth, and from the period of earliest infancy lives on within us. Because every psychotherapeutic setting allows the portrayal of certain connections better than others and even serves to hide some, only a multiple approach that shows the way in which pre- and perinatal experience actualizes in various forms of therapy can make the complexity of the situation clear. The following chapter contains a selection of case studies. It is hoped that through the sheer variety of the examples the reader will experience a significant expansion of his or her own powers of observation and openness to experience.

5

Restoring Health Through Reliving: The Actualization of Pre- and Perinatal Patterns of Behavior and Experience in Psychotherapy

THE APPEARANCE OF EARLY FORMS OF EXPERIENCE

To appreciate the following examples of the appearance of pre- and perinatal processes of experience, we must first address the significance of reliving in psychotherapy. We can picture human development as a series of developmental horizons—from embryo to fetus and newborn, followed by infant and small child, then child, teenager, and adult. Each developmental stage is a self-contained unit, a world of experiences unto itself. Later it is taken up into and transformed within the dynamic of the next developmental stage. Within this process, no experience is lost. We experience our

present circumstances in the light of experiences from
previous stages of our life. These experiences live on within
us albeit in our unconscious.

The transition from one developmental stage to the
next can go wrong because of traumatic experience. A
terrible experience that cannot be resolved remains uninte-
grated within the psyche and is not included in future
developments. The part of self-awareness that corresponds
to the trauma also remains undeveloped. Thus, in the
depths of the unconscious mind, one remains exactly the
child who suffered the trauma. In therapy this means that in
the case of early psychological damage the traumatizing
situation must be sought, and it is only through reenactment
that the small child, especially the one who has not yet
learned to speak, can deal with such wounds. I believe that
this is possible if psychoanalysts widen their perception for
preverbal dimensions of the individual unconscious. The
traumatic situation has to be played through once more in
order to treat it. This reliving and therapeutic repetition is
much more important for very early psychological wounds,
such as those from the pre- and perinatal period of life, than
for later traumatic events.

The wounding itself can affect various areas, for example leading to specific bodily sensations or to a specific
self-image. It can affect relationships and how one views life.
It can affect one's general mood and fantasy life. All of these
areas of experience, however, are woven together and can in
certain ways stand in for one another. An injury to the body
can persist on the physical level but it can also affect
relationships or show itself in particular dreams or private
fantasies. In fact a single traumatic injury can influence
various aspects of therapy and in so doing open itself to
treatment. This will be apparent in the case studies pre-

sented below. However, it is important to realize that the examples are relevant not only to psychotherapy. The therapeutic "staging" of the trauma has, in my opinion, a much greater value. What becomes quite apparent in the therapy also occurs in a similar fashion in other situations but is more concealed. Past events that have not been integrated in our psyche, especially those from the beginning of life, weave themselves into our life and experience. Our social and cultural organizations are influenced by our experiences at the beginning of our life. As will be later shown, these early experiences form a commonly shared background.

An important aspect of psychological injury causes a curious mixture of loss of memory (repression) and amplification of memory. Certain aspects of illnesses can remain almost photographically embedded in the memory while other aspects disappear almost completely. It is the same with preverbal memories. Distorted fragments are retained permanently in an intense memory and, although not understood, project themselves into our psychological life. So, for example, a particular gesture or a certain expression or bodily sensation can relate to a very early experience. Hackneyed expressions, repeated in all sorts of situations, for example, "banging my head against a brick wall," can be understood in connection with specific aspects of birth (Landsman 1989).

Early memories have a double-sided character: they are elusive and yet remain extremely present. Psychoanalysis has demonstrated this character for conflicts and injuries experienced by the small child. Making connections to the very earliest periods of life is still new and unusual for us. To help the reader to get a feel for the ways in which early experi-

ences show themselves, the results of various psychotherapies will now be discussed.

PRENATAL AND BIRTH EXPERIENCES AS SEEN IN PSYCHOANALYTIC THERAPY

In psychoanalysis, the significance of perinatal experiences
in therapy was discovered through the so-called date setting.
Freud (1966c) was analyzing a young man, whom he had
given the pseudonym "Wolfman," in reference to the patient's most important dream. The therapy had come to a
standstill and so Freud decided to get the therapeutic
process going again by setting a date by which the therapy
should be concluded. This procedure provoked what Otto
Rank later understood to have been an unconscious constel-
lation of birth. Apparently it produced a deep regression to
an earlier stage of development: "The patient gave the
impression of a lucidity which is normally only achieved in
hypnosis" (Freud 1966c, p. 34). The patient summarized his
suffering in a lamentation with the following content:

> The world was hidden from him by a veil. . . . The veil tore
> strangely enough only in one situation, namely, when his
> stool moved and passed through his anus as a result of an
> enema. Then he felt well again and for a very short time saw
> the world clearly. . . . Only shortly before the end of the
> treatment he remembered that he had heard that he had
> been born with a "Glückshaube" [amnion over his head]. [p.
> 132]

It was known that the Wolfman had suffered an eating
disorder as a baby. Then he had become ill, with almost fatal

consequences, when he was 3 months old. We know today that when someone has had such a difficult beginning to life, their earliest impressions are quite accessible to later consciousness and indeed can surface undisguised. Thus I presume that the world was really hidden from the Wolfman after his birth by the amniotic veil. We are dealing here with the phenomenon already mentioned of an intense memory of a traumatic episode. The Wolfman's constant state of anxiety and his fear of suffocation, which came out during the therapy, also point to a birth trauma. Such a connection is also confirmed by the relief from the memory of the birth trauma brought about by the symbolic repetition of birth— the enema. It is currently accepted in child psychotherapy that birth is symbolically repeated when bowel movement is accomplished. Just as in the case of the Wolfman, this allows pressure from the earlier bad experience to be released for a short time.

However, Freud himself did not come to these conclusions. Rather he interpreted the patient's complaint as the expression of a fantasy: "His complaint is actually the fulfilment of a fantasy desire. It shows him to have returned to his mother's womb, to be sure, the fantasy desire of fleeing from the world. It must be translated: 'I am so unhappy with life that I must return to my mother's womb'" (p. 134).

The decisive step taken by Otto Rank (1988) beyond this interpretation resulted from his conclusion that the fantasies were based on real experiences:

> The regular appearance of rebirth fantasies [at the end of therapy] can thus also be understood and their real basis becomes comprehensible in the analysis. The patient's "rebirth fantasies" prove themselves to be nothing less than

repetitions of his birth in the analysis, whereby the separation from the object of desire (libido), the analyst, seems to represent an exact reproduction of the first separation of the newborn from the first object of desire, the mother. The analysis turns out to be the belated disposal of the unresolved trauma of birth. [p. 26]

To make Rank's interpretation clear, I will now summarize several passages from a detailed report (1926) of one of his therapies. It concerns a middle-aged woman with a dependence problem who had had a difficult birth and who had then lost her mother when she was 12 years old. Her relationship to her father was not good.

In the fourth session, she reported that she had awoken from a dream which had ended as water engulfed her face. This dream is clearly a flight back to her (dead) mother before the analysis. She is even symbolised in the dream. The patient had added later that she had dreamt her mother had been lying on her back on a divan. The parallel is already clear here—analytical situation = womb situation. Of course, the patient was not informed of this.

20th session: "I was on a ship where we had to rehearse dances for some performance or other. In the process, I was grabbed by the feet and lying horizontally I was swung around violently in circles." Associations: "It is possible that I was somehow shaken in a similar way after my birth since I was later told that I had not breathed and some midwives used to let such children swing around by the legs a little with their head hanging downwards. By the way, I contracted whooping-cough even in my first year of life. The doctor said that was unusual. I was perhaps also somehow shaken around then in order to get me to breathe. I am a passionate dancer and had even as a child a lot of talent for it. I had an excellent feeling for rhythm and when I was eight years old could already dance very well. Yesterday I got a little dizzy because I had danced so much." After what has already been said, it is easy to see the significance of all this: the feeling in the dream combines the unpleasant birth trauma with the pleasant dance movements, that is, tries thereby to compensate. Since the patient also dates her dreams about obstructions and floating to her eighth year, then dancing was a motor displacement and sublimation of the same traumatic feelings.

In the 52nd session, she related she had woken up again exactly 5 minutes after 3:00 A.M. and could remember her dream. . . . Furthermore she reported a strange habit, actually a symptom. When she awakes in darkness, she gets up immediately to put the light on and then she falls unconscious again. Apparently, because she cannot stand the sudden light. . . . We can understand this symptom as well as her recent repression of dreaming when we hear that waking-up leads back to the light of dawn. . . . Now it seems obvious to us to see if the patient's intense birth trauma can provide an explanation here. When she saw the first glimmers of day-light, the light of the world so to speak, or when a light suddenly goes on in the dark, this reminds her of the first shock—which without doubt is also an intense optical one— and she can no longer sleep and so wakes up.

71st session: The patient related that she woke up again very early and had again dreamt of her father but did not know what. Afterwards she immediately fell asleep again and dreamt the following: "I was asleep in my room as someone came in and woke me up. I got up and went into the next room, looked at the wall and noticed that it was five past eleven. Thus I thought that I could not get to Dr. Rank on time. By the time I had got ready and got on my way, the time would be practically over. I should just tell him that I slept in and he would understand. Then I dreamt something about my father and then that I was travelling with lots of people on a ship which suddenly stopped. I thought we had set sail and now must wait until the flood comes. Then I felt that the ship was rocking and thought that we must still be moving. Then I wanted to disembark in a harbour but the pier was under water so that it was impossible to do so."

Interpretation: This dream shows clearly—as was said—to what extent the analyst had already begun to stand in for the father. . . . Thus this dream betrays the same tendency projected on the analyst to leave him waiting and not to come to the agreed appointment. . . . The reason why she cannot come to men is shown in the second dream sequence which clearly has the motif of fixation on the mother (lying in bed, ship) and which at the same time shows the significance to the analytical (mother) fixation in the contemporary situation. [pp. 63ff]

The quotations make it plain how in Rank's view early memories of real events are connected in a complex way to later fantasies and developmental needs and then in addition are interwoven with the actual relationship situation in the therapy. The therapist can only help the patient to overcome everything that prevents her happiness and stops her from finding her true identity when he is able to move freely back and forth between the various layers.

In 1924 Gustav Hans Graber published a book about the psychological significance of the change of environment that birth entails. He also tried later to communicate the background of his therapeutic experience in treatment reports. He emphasized how the prenatal stage of life can be the source of a strong desire to return to the womb. It can act like a shelter from the dangers of life. "It is the often unassailable and seemingly immutable resistance put up by the patient which paralyzes our efforts—their rigid, primal fixation, their regression to the embryonal state of existence with its demand for absolute security, god-like devotion, absolute generosity, etc." (Graber 1966, p. 93). Fear caused by birth trauma can be a decisive hindrance when it comes to taking real steps in life. The following example of treatment from Graber (1966) demonstrates this point:

A middle-aged academic stated that he had had the thought during his whole life that he really had not been born. He had felt always that he was in a prison which had no way out. As a consequence, he was stuck in a deep depression and had a disturbed relationship to the world and also to himself. Again and again a deep fear gripped him of going too far, a catastrophe which he experienced like a difficult birth. It was understandable that in the analysis he tried at first to hide in his shell. However, when he had recognised his intrauterine regression, he finally managed to activate a strong desire to free himself and was thus successful in getting himself moving in everyday life. [p. 182]

A therapy report from the Hungarian psychoanalyst Istvan Hollos also appeared in 1924. In it, he describes how a very early state of aggression experienced by a premature baby was reproduced with an almost uncanny precision during the course of therapy years later:

The first sentence which the patient spoke in the very first therapy session was: "I was born in the eighth month." . . . He lived convinced that he was physically and mentally inferior because he had been prematurely born. . . . After a short time in therapy, it became apparent that the patient's fantasies of self-destruction in which his self completely disintegrated into the tiniest particles was in fact intended to make a thorough and completely new birth possible, a birth

in which he would be born in full maturity at about nine
months. The attack (of chaotic rage and dissatisfaction)
was itself a symbolic self-destruction and destruction of his
parents. . . . The patient always had the fear of coming too
early, of acting prematurely. He could never be sure if
something was ready to be finished and got attacks (of rage
and grimacing) whenever he had come to the end of a piece
of work. He happily ripped up whole study books which he
had painstakingly written just when they were due to be
completed. . . . The cure began in February. On 16th April
the patient related the following dream: . . . "I was in
complete darkness where I continually drank blood. . . .
Suddenly it became clear to me that I was in the womb in
green water with a rope on my body. Suddenly something
began to push me out; it gradually became brighter. Then I
saw the room through the opening . . . the umbilical cord
had wrapped itself around my throat and was choking me just
as I had experienced in my attacks and after the injection and
I thought: Rather suffocation than cutting through the cord.
I pulled back. I did not want to be born at eight months
because of the cord. . . . However, it was too late. The cord
had been cut, the placenta began to detach itself. I almost fell
from the edge of the bed, I screamed and actually awoke
before 5 o'clock. It was already daylight and I recalled that I
had been born at this time. . . . Then the dream continued
though I was awake. I whimpered like a small child, just like
in my attacks, and I had the idea that I had urinated during
the birth. I had to get up and go to the toilet."

Through my contact with the patient and because of
the directness of some of the completely unusual expressions,
I became convinced that the presumption that this was a
case of make-believe or simulation could in no way fit the
facts. . . . The patient himself said that during his attacks he
could observe everything and knew everything and deliber-
ately allowed the gestures and behaviour led by instinct to

occur. He let the impulse which led to these outbreaks come over him. He wanted that "everything should come out" and he participated in the course of events taking place inside him with presence of mind and intellectual curiosity. He was trying to make sense of it all. . . . "I was born in the eighth month, too early. Just like the body, the psyche has also got to go through a normal process of development. Because I was born before this development was completed, this has left traces in my psyche and I have the idea that this is the reason why my unconscious cannot close. This defect has also got an advantage. It is thanks to this that I have not become mentally ill. Even during my attacks, the most important thing to me is that I always know what I am doing and do not hold myself back. One may think I am crazy but the main thing is that I keep myself in touch with normality [German here has 'with consciousness']." I must mention here that the cure went through particular phases and that the first, after which the attacks finally ceased, came to an end after nine months. The patient had really revisited the womb between February and October and had then gone through a rebirth and had made up for the missing ninth month. [pp. 423–433]

At the end of the 1940s, Nandor Fodor, an analyst also of Hungarian origin, published several works about manifestations of birth and how to deal with them in psychoanalysis. He gave examples of very precise reproductions in dreams and in therapy sessions:

In the fourth session of her analysis, Ivette said: "I dreamt that I was a small baby and somebody or other was hitting me on my bare back. This gave me a terrible shock. I was very small, no bigger than a doll, and the shock was like flames of light which shot into my brain. This confused and surprised me. I did not have any feeling of pain at the time and I did not cry."

The analysis of the dream then led to a reliving of birth sensations:

"I have a strange feeling in my legs. I feel weak and fall down. I have a sinking feeling, an unpleasant feeling. I am dozy as if under anesthetic. My head is bent backwards and I am moving backwards. I feel like I am being born. It is a little difficult and I make some effort with my legs. It is a completely normal position. My head is to one side and I shoot backwards. I feel frightened. Then the fear is gone." Her head was leaning to the side and was half over the edge of the couch. She pulled herself straight again and sighed: "It is terribly exhausting—this birth business." [1949, pp. 78ff]

A report from the Swiss psychoanalyst Stefan Blarer (1982) brings this series of case studies to a close. It concerns a 26-year-old psychology student who suffered from the inability to make friends and especially to form relationships with women:

As soon as he becomes even slightly nervous, a tick starts up whereby the patient must stop the flow of air in his throat at short intervals. He gets very angry with himself for doing so. Whenever he embraces a girl, he gets the feeling that he is being strangled by something invisible. For a long time he was unable to follow my suggestion to lie down on the couch because he was frightened that his feelings would choke him. In the course of analysis, at the so-called seams in the therapy, when a breakthrough was on its way, he always brought dreams with the same pattern: "I come from a passage into light. I glide to the ground with a parachute but I break right though the surface and hang in empty space above Hell. . . . Brightness penetrates my eyes and then it goes dark. A mouth approaches me in order to bite my head off.—Then it turns

me to the left with force and I would rather go to the right."
The mother related (later) that the patient was born earlier
than expected at home. Just as he was already a little bit out,
the birth did not continue because the umbilical cord was
wrapped around his neck. A doctor was immediately called
but it took about half-an-hour until the birth could be
brought to an end. [pp. 122ff]

The California psychoanalyst Lynda Share (1994, 1996)
has recently opened new pathways in our understanding of
early preverbal material in the psychoanalytic situation by
means of a new way of interpreting dreams based on the
work of the Los Angeles psychoanalyst Bernard Bail. Important in this context was her clarification of the old discussion
between those psychoanalysts who believed that psychoanalysis is narrative in respect to early experiences, and those who
believed that early experiences are retained in an individual's memory. Her conclusion is that there are two memory
systems, one verbal and linked to the narrative level, and the
other a primitive preverbal memory system linked to memo-
rizing through reenactment and symbolizing in images and
symptoms. In her book *If Someone Speaks It Gets Lighter:
Dreams and the Reconstruction of Infant Trauma*, she gives many
impressive examples of her way of interpreting dreams by
integrating the early preverbal level of experience. She
shows that it is possible to understand certain dreams as
telling a story of real preverbal experiences.

Another recent initiative to integrate the prenatal dimension in psychoanalysis comes from Brazilian psychoanalyst Joanna Wilheim (1992, 1995). Based on Bion, she
proposes taking the prenatal development from conception
to birth as a basic matrix of unconscious fantasies. She
assumes, for example, that the basic matrix of feelings of

rejection and acceptance is shaped at conception and implantation. In this understanding anguish is rooted in early prenatal experiences of real threats to life or losing the providing and containing object. It is to be hoped that these new ideas will become the subject of more general discussion.

An especially good starting point for such a discussion could be the clinical and empirically orientated articles of Philadelphia psychoanalyst John C. Sonne (1994a,b, 1996). Sonne presents clinical material from psychoanalytic sessions that shows how deep anxieties can be rooted in the prenatal experience of the dread of abortion. He shows as well how interpreting these connections can help patients integrate these wounding experiences.

In Germany, too, a discussion on the prenatal dimension in psychoanalysis is slowly emerging (Janus 1988, 1989b). Child analysts in particular are active in this field and demonstrate how perinatal states of emergency are reenacted in the therapeutic play (Friedrich 1993, 1996, Hungar 1996, Kugele 1990, Leyh 1996, Schier 1993, Storch 1991). Adult therapists are also beginning to describe their experiences with early preverbal reenactments in the psychoanalytic situation (Blazy 1991b, Eschenbach 1994, Gsell 1995, Huber 1994, 1995, Janus 1990b,d, 1994, Reiter 1995, Schindler 1983).

It is interesting that the subject of perinatal experiences in the history of psychoanalysis was occasionally mentioned in the discussion, but never taken seriously, because it appeared to be in contradiction to common sense. It should be mentioned that such influential psychoanalysts as Greenacre (1945), Heimann (1989), and Winnicott (1988, 1992) took the enduring effects of the birth experience for granted and believed them to be an important issue in therapy, but they did not systematize this insight.

With this background, it is possible to reread Freud's case histories to see whether there are also pre- and perinatal images, as I have done in the cases of Little Hans and Dora (Janus 1991e).

REPORTS OF PRENATAL AND BIRTH MEMORIES IN HYPNOSIS

In comparison with previous epochs, it is now easier for us to recognize that memories of prenatal and early postnatal states can reveal themselves under hypnosis. Even reflexes from the early phases of life can become operative again (Raikov 1980).

Various insights into the psychology of early experiences had already been expressed in the nineteenth century and the area was also discussed in detail by the first psychoanalysts. These early developments have recently been surveyed by Terence Dowling (1991a).

It was not known that hypnosis is essentially determined by the reactivation of pre- and early postnatal states of consciousness. This is because the focus was on the techniques of induction and the effects of the altered state of awareness they produce. Because hypnosis can reactivate such early experiences, hypnotherapists have been the ones in a position to report very impressive examples of the retrieval of pre- and perinatal memories.

It has been observed that the head and shoulder movements that occur during the process of birth can spontaneously appear again in hypnotically induced age regression (Cheek 1974). Comparison with reports about the actual birth produced quite amazing and almost 100 percent agreement. By this technique, complaints that can be related back to birth trauma, such as migraine, neck muscle tension, and asthma attacks, can be resolved in a single session. Elements of the birth can be actualized in painful bodily experiences with exceptional precision. Also experiences of prenatal bliss or fear that can be brought into consciousness during hypnosis can be proven to have been authentic by objective research carried out later. This demonstrates that the pre- and perinatal abilities of the child to perceive and comprehend what happens to him or her are far more complex than has been previously imagined. The experimental research of the developmental psychologist Anthony DeCasper (DeCasper and Fifer 1980), concerning the recognition of prenatal memory traces, indicates something of the complexity of a baby's perceptual abilities before birth to become clear.

Let us for the moment ponder the often astonishing reports of the memory's ability under hypnosis. The hypnotherapist Claus Bick (1986) reports the following case:

> The twenty-five-year-old Renata Sch. suffered from terrible states of anxiety, depression and hot flushes. Under hypnosis, she was brought back into the womb. While she was reliving the period about three months before her birth, her heart suddenly began to race, she experienced a strong hot flush and shouted: "All my problems began with this feeling!" Then she began to cry and said that it was gradually getting hotter and thought that hot water had something to do with it. And this water made her frightened: "It is getting hotter. I cannot stand it any longer. My heart is bursting!" I led her back one month further—then there were no problems. A further three months regression—again no problems. After completing the hypnosis and bringing the patient back into a state of normal consciousness, one suspicion was obvious: attempted abortion. A telephone call to her mother confirmed it: after

a little hesitation, the mother admitted that she had tried several times during the pregnancy to abort Renata. To do so, she had, among other things, taken hot hip-baths. [p. 109]

The following report is about a patient who suffered from severe headaches and attacks of anxiety and depression:

Under hypnosis, she experienced herself again and again with headaches: in school, playing in a meadow, where she would suddenly hold her aching head. Only when she was led back into the womb, did she become free of the complaint. Then we looked at her birth. Suddenly the woman shouted: "My head!" In answer to my question: "What is wrong with your head?", she replied: "It is falling. It has fallen on the floor!"—"Is nobody there?"—"No!"—"Have you got headaches?" I asked spontaneously. She answered, "Yes, I have just got headache."

Questioning of the mother shed light on the matter. The mother had canned a lot of pears and had eaten a huge amount of them. She thought that there was still a bit of time before the baby was due. When she felt pressure in her belly on the following day, she thought that it must be the pears and that she had better go to the toilet. However, she did not even get as far as that. In her fear, she pulled a bucket from the cupboard and then followed the daughter's unexpected and extraordinary birth. After this experience had been sorted out, the headaches never returned. [p. 111]

The experience of a traumatic birth as relived under hypnosis was described as follows. During the analysis of her birth, the patient reported experiencing fear and continued:

"It is so dark, I want to get out, I want to get out. My mother resists, she is frightened. She is frightened because she is alone. She holds me in and shouts for someone. It is so dark, I want to get out. It is so dark, I am frightened. I am frightened and I want to get out. Please let me out!" She began to scream and cry. Inquiry afterwards confirmed that the mother had been alone at the time of the birth and that the father was on his way to fetch the midwife. She continued then: "It is so terrible, I am falling, I am falling. I am shivering so much." Her answer to the question as to where she now was led to the idea that she had been a precipitate delivery. [p. 193]

Many protocols from hypnosis therapy record that the child before birth can perceive that their parents quarrel or reject them. This fact is confirmed in reports from experiences in LSD therapy, which will be discussed in more detail later. There are also dramatic portrayals of loneliness after birth, an experience that can form the basis of later feelings of abandonment.

REACTIVATION OF BIRTH MEMORIES IN PRIMAL THERAPY

Arthur Janov developed his primal therapy out of his observation that patients can spontaneously experience a very deep regression when they are appropriately supported. An important element of the primal scream therapy is the repetition again and again of aspects of the birth, the so-called birth primals. As an example, here are some passages from a report (1984) about a patient who was a breech birth:

From the very beginning of the primal experience, the patient complained about feeling that his legs and backside were cold—and the patient's skin actually did feel cold. At intervals of a few seconds, he doubled up and was seized by spasms. However, he could not understand what was happening to him. . . . "My body was twitching like crazy and I had all sorts of pains especially in my back. My groaning, it was like fighting so that I would not be crushed. . . . I have a feeling of pressure spreading from a point a little above my backside up to my armpits—I feel the worst pain a little under my shoulder-blades because I have got my hands folded in front of me. . . . My body is cold below and above warm. It seems as though I am split in the middle and because of this the upper part of my body is in pain. . . . It is as if my backbone is being twisted and as if strong muscles are crushing me. . . . I have pain in the right shoulder. I do not know what it means but it is as if I am being gripped in a chute and as if someone is contorting my body and twisting my shoulders. And everything is tearing my back out. [p. 321]

The resumé of the patient's pattern of life provides us with some striking information:

"During my whole life I was always on the point of getting involved in a fight with someone who had hit me or even just provoked me. At school I always reacted too strongly when some child or other pushed me by accident and then it came to a brawl. Now I realise that I have always been defending myself against these early pains. Everything that today causes me pain sets my birth pain free and then I have to strike out in order to protect myself from further pain." [p. 326]

This statement shows how such early traumatic memories can lie just under the surface of everyday life and, without us knowing, influence our behavior.

The following report from the German primal therapist Klaus Bieback (1991) concerns a 22-year-old woman whose development to adult maturity was hindered by archaic fears:

It is known from the biography of this woman that her mother who was on a holiday-trip at the time had nearly lost her baby in the third month of pregnancy—she had begun to bleed. The cervix had opened to 25 millimetres and the hospital doctor at first believed this to be the result of an attempted abortion—which was not the case. The mother had to remain lying down for five days and was not allowed to move. The doctors said that the chances of success were not higher than 5 percent. She was given Valium and her vital functions became very slow. The bleeding stopped. A healthy child was then born after a further six months of normal pregnancy.

The woman's early frightening experience is reflected in the following strange dream:

"My younger sister had been sent to help me by my father: there was a high mountain like a cone. It is like a pyramid and its walls are as smooth as mirrors. Our car is standing right at the top on a platform. The platform is just big enough for the tyres to fit on so that the car protrudes over the edges and is about to slip off. My father is behind the wheel with his sister sitting next to him. Mother and I are outside. I then had to tell father how he had to drive, first a little forwards, then a little backwards. It is a matter of millimetres. I cannot bear to look. It is a matter of life or death. I have full responsibility although I actually don't want it and can't cope. For a long time, it hangs in the balance. Then it is over. I was forced to do it but nothing bad happened and it is over and done with. But then the same thing begins to happen again at the back. The car is on a vertical, slippery wall and only the front tyres are holding it on the platform. I have to control everything so that it does not go so quickly. Everything very, very slowly. Actually, it is impossible. There could be a crash. The car has to stand vertically and can only move millimetre by milli-

metre. Otherwise it would not have enough hold. It would have crashed and exploded.—Then I woke up."
    I would like here to give the dream a title, the same one that I gave to the woman. It reads: "Life before the crash had right of way—very, very slowly." Then I continued: "You and the car managed magnificently. Congratulations." She looked at me, surprised and grateful. She and I knew that I had visited her on her dangerous mountain. With the positive outcome in view, the integration of the traumatic experience could be begun and continued. [p. 74]

This report makes it clear how symbolic "derivatives" of a prenatal trauma can present themselves in dreams and in psychotherapeutic communication. The revival and subsequent handling of these derivatives is necessary if adult independence is to be achieved. The preverbally centered psychotherapeutic setting takes on a particular importance in the very effective psychotherapy of babies with pre- or perinatal traumatization (Emerson 1989, 1996).

REACTIVATION OF PERINATAL TRAUMA IN PSYCHOANALYTIC REGRESSION THERAPY

In more recent forms of psychotherapy, there have been various attempts to unite elements of psychoanalysis, primal therapy, and body-oriented therapy to create for patients an optimal psychotherapeutic setting in which to relive early traumatic experiences. An example of this is the psychoanalytic regression therapy developed by the psychoanalyst Wolfgang Hollweg (1995). I quote his report (1990) of the treatment of a 9-year-old girl who suffered from an inexplicable rheumatic condition in her legs:

I encouraged her (in the first therapy session) to lie on the
floor, to keep her eyes tight closed and to concentrate as hard
as she could on the pain in her legs. She should then tell me
what she could feel in her body. After a few minutes, she
began to laugh. "I want to make a somersault." I encouraged
her to follow her instinct. She then made several somersaults,
one after the other. Suddenly she stopped and said: "It is no
longer possible. I have to make a somersault but it is far too
cramped to do so!" Her voice sounded now completely
different. She sounded tense and frightened. Finally she said:
"I am stuck in a very small room. I must get out head first but
I am lying the wrong way round. I cannot turn!" [p. 57]

In the next session the girl experienced her birth. She
was a so-called "breech birth." She was able to give a very
satisfactory explanation of how her birth-position was connected to the fears which always came over her when she went
to the toilet. In a toilet, she is just unable to free herself from
the thought that a hand could come up and grab her buttocks
and pull her down. She could see the connection between
this and the events of her birth quite clearly and she was able
to resolve quite a lot of the fear bound up with the situation.

After this phase, she saw herself back in the womb in the
last months of the pregnancy. She was lying the wrong way
round with her buttocks downwards and with her legs pulled
up so that her feet were pressed against her mother's
abdominal wall. She could feel how an enormous pressure
coming from her feet was pressing her knees and lower legs.
She experienced it as so painful that she could hardly sleep or
relax in the womb. An experience occurred a few sessions
later which uncovered the cause of her breech position. At
first, she heard the noise of a car motor. Then suddenly she
perceived, together with this noise, the sound of brakes
screeching and then a violent jolt. Then she felt as if she had
been flung out. Only after this was she lying the wrong way.
Up until this event, she had been in the correct position for

birth. What had happened? The mother had taken driving lessons during the pregnancy even in the ninth month. Once when she had pulled the brakes on too hard, the baby turned. The therapy demonstrated that she had tried afterwards to correct her wrong position but she had been unable because there was just less and less room. The therapy was cut short at this point because after this experience, the symptoms quickly cleared up. The girl was able to go to high school without any problems. [p. 57]

The report is so plausible that it needs hardly any comment. It clearly shows that a person in a conflict situation can spontaneously revert to behavior connected with a much earlier trauma. This fact is very easy to overlook and one must learn from experience how to recognize this regressive tendency of our normal, everyday experience and behavior. When that is possible, then it is much easier to make real connections between such fears as the toilet anxiety that plagued Hollweg's patient and the experience of birth. The following principle can be formulated: Our whole experience of life, including our pre- and perinatal experiences, remains active within us. Our experience of birth, our first experience of change and transformation, can become active and influence the course in a supportive or negative way of any quick process of change in our later life as adolescent or adult.

VISUALIZATION OF PRE- AND PERINATAL EVENTS UNDER THE INFLUENCE OF LSD

There is a comprehensive literature about the effects of LSD. However, this includes very little about the reliving of pre-

and perinatal primal experiences. Only very few authors, such as Hanscarl Leuner, Stanislaw Grof, Ralf Bolle, and Athanassios Kafkalides have made systematic investigations of the ability of LSD to activate early memories. LSD belongs to the so-called psychoactive substances that provoke an experience of the normally unconscious contents of the deep psyche. This occurs in the form of a sort of intense daydream. During the 1960s and 1970s some, for example members of subcultures, hoped that an enhanced consciousness could be achieved with the help of LSD. However, it was quickly evident that a destabilization of the personality occurred in people with a neurotic disposition and that the way toward regression and addiction was opened. Nevertheless, LSD remains, when it is applied in a controlled way, a useful instrument for research of the deep unconscious.

Here is a typical example of an experience under LSD reported by the American birth specialist, Leni Schwartz (1983):

> After twenty minutes I began to feel the effect of the drug. . . . The spiral form with which I had identified myself transformed itself into a dark, cavelike room. I felt its boundaries. . . . I began to move myself slowly down a long tunnel. The walls bulged rhythmically in and out. They were made of a damp material which was making pulsating, contracting and expanding movements. At the end of the tunnel, there was a blue light. . . . Like the blue sky of a beautiful, spring day. . . . Suddenly everything changed. I felt an unbearable pressure on my head and body, a terrible pain. I was being pushed backwards by an overpowering force but it was impossible to move forward. Instead, the soft walls got narrower. All movement stopped. I was trapped, near to

suffocation and too small and powerless to fight against the unexpected force. With a frightened scream, in a mixture of anger and fear, I heard myself shouting: "Help me, I am too small, I cannot breathe, I cannot manage it alone. Why have you left me alone, where are you? I need you." For a time that seemed to me to be neverending, I felt near to death—alone, abandoned, in a dark cage without air. There was no exit, I could not go forwards or backwards. Then, just as unexpectedly as the movements had stopped, they began again. The pulsating was intense and rhythmical. I began to fight in earnest and to work my way forwards. I wept and cried often because of the pain. . . . Then the battle suddenly stopped and I broke out of my prison into a place of clear blue light. This expulsion was accompanied by an intense pain in my neck. I gasped for air. . . . I was exhausted but free. [p. 19]

Schwartz describes in a very convincing way how she was able as a result of this impressive birth experience under LSD to find many connections to her basic feelings and attitudes toward life. She often experienced fears of being left alone and loss of courage, which could now be understood in connection to her birth. Small disappointments often led her to dramatic feelings of having been left alone. She had always tried in every conceivable way to avoid being left alone. "Now I try to connect this feeling with what I know about my birth." After talking with her mother, she was also able to make other connections between what she had experienced under LSD and real events.

It is clear that the LSD does not create completely original and new experiences but only brings aspects of the deep unconscious into the light of consciousness. Through a systematic comparison of the various types of experience produced by LSD, it was possible to see that certain fundamental perinatal experiences had had a special influence.

They had formed basic structures in the mind that then influenced the person's pattern of experience in later life. Grof named these deep structures "matrices," by which he meant that the various stages of birth—the prenatal phase, the phases of cervical opening, of expulsion and finally of delivery—mould basic psychological structures that influence later experience. These basic experiences form the foundation, the background, and point of departure for later experiences of life and coming to terms with the world.

If the pattern of the matrices contains distortions as a result of Grof's subjective standpoint, one must remember it is the same with all first attempts. Nevertheless, they must be seen to represent a conceptual breakthrough in the psychodynamic registration of the basic, pre- and perinatal patterns of experience. The systematic distortions are due to an underestimation of prenatal trauma or, put another way, an overestimation of the "good womb." The creative and productive elements of the birth struggle are also underestimated and the aspects of death and destruction valued too highly. As a result, Grof tends to see a definite split between a "good," primal experience in the womb and a "bad" experience of death during birth. He also mythologizes the whole experience to a certain extent. Nevertheless, if one does not forget the above-mentioned distortions, the system of perinatal matrices is a very useful concept. It helps in the consideration and categorization of early experience. I will therefore present in summary form aspects of the various stages of pre- and perinatal experience according to Grof (1988, pp. 117–171).

Basic Perinatal Matrix I (BPM I)—
Primal Union with the Mother

Life in the womb is "connected with a state of blissful, undifferentiated, oceanic consciousness." Test subjects had the feeling of "being one with their environment" and of "being united with the object they were perceiving."

The test subjects reported having very distinct memories under LSD of irritation experienced during their prenatal life, for example, those caused by the mother being physically or psychologically burdened. These can consist of optical disturbances, such as being wrapped in fog, or they can be expressed in specific physical symptoms such as headache, feeling weak, or being cold. Also "visions of demons" or "angry deities" that occurred in some experiments point to crises experienced before birth.

Basic Perinatal Matrix II (BPM II)—Fighting Against the
Mother (Contractions in a Closed Uterine System)

This stage corresponds to the first clinical stage of birth. This is physically a situation of great distress and threat, full of pain and constriction. "The test subjects felt themselves to be trapped in a claustrophobic world and experienced unbelievable physical and psychological agony." Not even the thought of suicide seemed to be comforting here. Pictures of Hell and unending torment came up. Ideas about disgusting and misformed beings also occurred. "The agony of birth is identical with the agony of death." The destiny of mythological figures like Sisyphus, Tantalus, or Prometheus are put forward as illustrations of this experience of torment as is also the expulsion from paradise or the crucifixion of Jesus Christ. "An intensification of the experience typically leads to a vision of a gigantic, irresistible whirlpool, a cosmic maelstrom, which mercilessly sucks the afflicted person and his world into itself." The typical bodily symptoms that occur when this phase is being remembered are extreme pressure on the head and body, ringing in the ears, breathing and heart difficulties, alternating hot and cold flushes.

Basic Perinatal Matrix III (BPM III)—Working with the Mother (Moving Forward Through the Birth Canal)

"The test subject experiences a series of immense compressions of energy and then their explosive discharge and expresses the feeling that powerful streams of energy are flowing through his whole body." These experiences are often accompanied by visions of natural catastrophes: earthquakes, volcanic eruptions, floods and storms of biblical proportions. But also sadomasochistic imaginings and general sexual excitement go together with these memories. The observation that boys can have an erection at birth fits with this.

Basic Perinatal Matrix IV (BPM IV)—Separation from the Mother (Ending of the Symbiotic Unity and Formation of a New Form of Relationship)

Suddenly, after the distressing torment, the test subject feels "relief and relaxation." Sometimes, very precise memories of these last events of the birth are produced, memories that seem to be confirmed when independent witnesses are asked: the smell of anesthetics, the rattling of medical instruments, light, but also specific medical interventions such as use of forceps or efforts to resuscitate.

> After the person has experienced the worst, total destruction
> and has reached the cosmic abyss, he is then assaulted by
> visions of blinding white or golden light. . . . The receptivity
> towards natural beauty is greatly increased and a simple,
> uncomplicated life in close contact with nature seems to be
> the most desirable form of existence. . . . Probably the
> symbolic frame of reference which appears most frequently
> for this experience is the death of Christ on the Cross and his
> Resurrection, the Mystery of Good Friday and the Revelation
> of the Holy Grail. [pp. 117–175]

The astonishing profusion of images and connections
produced by these experiments with drugs may be strange
and stir criticism. In spite of this, fundamental elements of
early experience—elements that are normally seen only in
very incomplete and modified forms in our social and
cultural life—are described here. In this sense, images
produced under drugs do make our earliest experiences
present again.

The long-term effects of prenatal experience upon the
life and feelings of an adult can become quite clearly
apparent under LSD. The Greek psychiatrist and psychotherapist Athanassios Kafkalides (1995) has developed here
the concept of the *accepting* and of the *rejecting womb*. To
illustrate the influence of a rejecting womb, here is an
example from Kafkalides. It concerns a 20-year-old, single
woman who has felt like a frightened animal ever since her
childhood. She is frightened of everything and cannot find
support anywhere. She feels only guilt within herself and
punishes and torments herself because of these feelings.
Here are extracts from the protocol of the LSD-experience:

> As I saw my mother pregnant, I felt that I was in her belly and
> that she was hitting me dreadfully. It became clear to me that

she wanted to abort me and I felt frightened because everyone was against me and I felt very weak. . . . The womb is
something unclean. It contains paper rubbish and broken
glass. When someone manages to get in there, he ceases to
exist. It is like a grave, like being in a plastic bag. . . . I
cannot see the sea because it is drowning me. And as I am
drowning, I become a small baby, a fetus, and then . . . then
the grave is there. . . . And if I did not exist in the womb,
how could I believe that I have ever existed? . . . I feel
permanently dead and permanently defend myself. . . .
When will I get out of this situation? . . . It is black. I come
out naked and people do not like others who are naked. I feel
as though I am burning . . . I can see black ash . . . What
is it? The womb is everywhere. I enter the world as if I have
been burned. After my birth, I have come out of the womb
but I cannot resist it because everywhere I am I feel as if I am
still inside of it. I have the feeling that I have always got the
womb around me even though I am outside of it. . . . I am
still the small, dirty child that they did not want. [pp. 21ff]

In such reports as this, the terrible misery caused by the
earliest form of rejection becomes clear. This misery can be
hidden behind oppressive fear and feelings of inferiority.
For this patient there was only a terrible, life-denying lesson
to be learned. Marie Cardinal has described in her book *Les
mots pour le dire* (1979) how such a lesson can be reflected in
a more psychoanalytically oriented therapy process.

From a neurophysiological point of view, the plethora of
images produced by LSD corresponds to increased activity of
the right cerebral hemisphere, the area of the brain more
concerned with the processing of images. The left hemisphere processes the more abstract and linguistic information. At the same time, this represents a pattern of brain
activity that is like that of the child or infant. Thus, psy-

cholytic substances probably cause a neurologically determined form of regression and an activation of early layers of experiences.

BIRTH EXPERIENCES IN REBIRTHING

Leonard Orr, the founder of rebirthing, recognized as a result of personal experience the great significance of a raised breathing rhythm as a means of returning to early states of experiences. He discovered that it was possible to encourage regression by breathing more quickly like babies do.

This is nothing other than the rediscovery in the West of the expansion of consciousness possible by altered and intensified breathing, the so-called circular breathing without pausing between inhalation and exhalation, known and practiced in the East and Near East for centuries. It is remarkable that the effects of circular breathing were discovered simultaneously in several different Western countries. However, Orr was the most persuasive advocate of this new technique of altering consciousness. The regression can reach various depths, especially perinatal and very early postnatal stages. This is probably because perinatal respiratory distress is relatively frequent and because the altered breathing in rebirthing seems to activate just such memories and such perinatal bodily conditions. Here is an example of rebirthing from the therapist Wolfgang Strasser (1988):

> In my second session, a very important part of my birth experience came up. I had the feeling of slowly but surely drifting towards a dark chasm and that I could not get away from this chasm. This made me very frightened that I was

going to die. This experience evidently corresponded to the
phase of being constricted during the process of birth. A
second manifestation of my birth only occurred much later,
in fact in the thirtieth session. In this second "birth session,"
I experienced at first a really beautiful, calm breathing
rhythm and everything was natural and harmonious. But
slowly I felt how an enormous pressure on my body, especially
on my left side, became gradually stronger and stronger so
that I almost couldn't stand it any longer. . . . After a while,
this pressure decreased and it became brighter around me. I
began to freeze, my whole body was shivering and my teeth
were really chattering. A feeling of deep loneliness came over
me. However, the worst thing which I had to fight against was
the impression that my consciousness was slowly but surely
disappearing. . . . On the one side, I thought to myself that
this must have been a part of my birth experience and that my
birth must have involved great difficulty. After my birth, I
evidently did not know if I was going to survive it all.
(According to reports of people who were present at my
birth, it had been in fact quite complicated.) Then the
assistant came and simply laid my hands on my body and on
my head and in a flash I felt very much better. I could relax
better and knew that I was not alone in the world. After a few
minutes I was suddenly certain that I did not have to
die. . . . It was as if I had received the gift of life again. Then
I became incredibly hungry. With the hunger, all the previous
drastic experiences slowly receded and I came back to myself.
[p. 92]

It is possible, as already mentioned, that rebirthing
activates especially experiences that occurred directly after
birth. In any case, rebirthers have made special contribu-
tions here. To use the expression of Terence Dowling, the
whole psychosomatic configuration of a person's birth can

be called his or her "birth script." Such birth scripts, which are composed of somatic, psychological, and relationship experiences, can have a marked effect on later development. This is especially the case when these scripts cannot be adequately dealt with in the postnatal mother–child interaction. They can then be expressed in fixed patterns of behavior and lead to frequently repeated scenes. Examples of such scripts are: "I must try harder." "Everything is a fight!" "I am guilty." "I am pulled back and forth." "I am powerless." "I cannot find any way out." "I am wounded." "I cannot get through." "I must suddenly look after myself."

This is only a partial expression of the birth script. One can observe how certain aspects of one's own birth script can be repeated and played out in particular social interactions. This can be understood as an attempt to integrate the experiences. However, very often it is simply the expression of a limited approach to life and to oneself, the limits having been set by early experiences, especially birth. Patterns of behavior that are permanently repeated throughout life are very often the blind repetition of experiences made at birth. Examples of this are commitment anxiety, compulsive dependence, flight from relationship, masochistic or sadistic conflicts, inability to separate and protect oneself in a destructive relationship, repeatedly arriving too early or too late.

As the examples from the use of LSD demonstrated, various states of suffering and danger can be revived by a deep regression and these states can very easily go beyond the individual's ability to deal with them. As a result of this, the torments of birth are very often averted and blocked by idealizing prenatal existence. The womb is then seen as a paradise, an ideally good place to live. The rebirthing movement exemplifies the danger of belief in utopian healing and healing communities. Fear leads to a sort of mythological short-circuit and a grasping at certainty and security. The sobering reality, however, is that there is still a massive amount of research to be carried out in the area of pre- and perinatal psychology. At the moment, we have only crude guesses and first impressions. There is far more uncertainty and many more unanswered questions than definitive knowledge.

THE SIGNIFICANCE OF EARLY EXPERIENCE IN OTHER FORMS OF PSYCHOTHERAPY

The examples and the discussion in this chapter may enable the reader to make connections to his or her own experience and to uncover and decipher a part of one's own early biography. Perhaps as a result the reader has been able to see through one's projections and gain a better awareness of oneself, an expansion of one's consciousness. The same thing can happen among friends and acquaintances who are interested in trying to understand the importance of life's beginning. Surprising connections between early experience and present behavior and attitude to life can arise and lead to a deeper self-understanding. Only an enhanced self-awareness and a better appreciation of one's attitude to life can offer real access to the biographical significance of our earliest experiences. For this reason, the following chapter is concerned with further, empirical observations of the long-term effects of pre- and perinatal influences.

6

The Perils of Birth: Empirical Findings About the Effects of Pre- and Perinatal Stress

The long-term effects of pre- and perinatal stress can be studied in various ways, and a number of comprehensive reports have been published. There is a particular problem in this area, which needs to be addressed immediately. There is no question that there is enough evidence for what can be called a *prenatal stress syndrome*. It generally appears postnatally in the prenatally stressed individual as a reduced resistance to stress or an increased irritability.

The problem lies in the common reluctance to think about these problems. Perhaps it raises disquieting questions about the circumstances of one's own early life or begins to confront us with some feelings of helplessness that we experienced during our own birth. Perhaps it threatens the commonsense discretion that protects us from the frightening and threatening effects of approaching any personal fear. However, if we overcome our reluctance, the new knowledge about the significance of the earliest traumatic experiences in our life can help us to cope better with all sorts of problems, and it begins to make prevention of problems possible.

PRENATAL STRESS IN ANIMALS

As early as the 1950s, the American researcher William R. Thompson (1957) convincingly demonstrated that the offspring of rat mothers that had been stressed when they were pregnant were behaviorally disturbed and remained so even until the end of their lives. The rats showed a permanently increased level of anxiety. Thompson assumed that the maternal stress had been communicated to the unborn rats by her stress hormones, hormones that also cross the placenta in humans. A further significant finding was that the effects of the stress were seen to be retained in the family and transmitted for several generations (Ward and Ward 1989). Not only were the female rats that had been prenatally stressed less fertile, with more spontaneous abortions, vaginal bleeding, and longer pregnancies, but even their offspring, that is the grandchildren of the rat that had been originally stressed when she was pregnant, were less viable and had decreased birth weight. More recent research has not only confirmed the increased anxiety levels in prenatally stressed rats but has also found that the prenatal stress changes the dopamine activity in their brains (Peters 1988; for a literature survey, see Cullen and Connolly 1987,

Janus and Maiwald 1992, Maiwald 1994, Maiwald and Janus 1993).

There is considerable evidence that another effect of prenatal stress observed in animals also occurs in humans. Prenatal stress leads to a feminization of male individuals. This occurs because the prenatal stress influences the levels of androgen hormone, which in turn influences the sexually specific development of the brain (see Dörner 1988). However, it is interesting that many of the behavioral disturbances caused by prenatal stress can be diminished by special care and intensive skin contact after birth. This confirms the observation already mentioned that the effects of pre- and perinatal trauma in humans can be minimized by good postnatal care.

Postnatal neuropsychological sensitivity shows itself in the fact that experimental animals can be negatively or positively influenced for the rest of their lives by the way in which they are treated after birth. Behavioral disturbances are caused in rats that are separated from their mothers after their birth. Humans seem to be quite similar in this regard: children who have suffered separation from their mother and/or neglect early in their lives perform and behave less well in school.

PRENATAL AND BIRTH STRESS IN HUMANS

This area of research is so large that it can only be presented here in summary form. The extreme loss of security for pregnant mothers during times of war provides an opportunity to study the effects of stress on human reproduction on a very large scale. The developmental psychologist Lester Sontag (1944) was the first to do this. He reported that children conceived during the alarming conditions of war had an increased heart rate in the womb and a decreased birth weight. Furthermore, an increased heart rate and increased irritability could be observed even years later in adulthood. These observations inspired the gynecologist Antonio Ferreira (1960) to make a statistical study of the significance of the mother's attitude to her unborn child. This study showed conclusively that the babies had been strongly affected by their mother's negative and fearful attitude toward them in the womb.

Such studies then encouraged the psychologist Gerhard Rottmann (1974) to carry out a longitudinal study in which the behavior and psychological state of the pregnant mother were clearly seen to determine in a statistically significant way the condition of her newborn baby. The more conflict, ambivalence, and rejection the mother demonstrated in her relationship with her unborn child, the more the child was affected after its birth. The more balanced the mother and positively oriented toward her child, the more adjusted was her newborn child. An extensive review of the existing studies enabled the psychoanalyst Theodor Hau (1982) to summarize the effects of prenatal stress upon the condition of the baby in the following sentences:

1. Less sleep, increased unquietness and irritability, disturbances of perception and attention.
2. In later development: disturbances in the formation of concepts, decreased verbal, ideational and general IQ.
3. Excessive screaming, apathy and/or states of extreme restlessness.
4. Underweight and weight loss, disturbances of food intake, gastrointestinal disturbances. [p. 36]

The strong reaction of the unborn child to stress can no longer be questioned. The plethora of anecdotal accounts, many of them now well known, serve to popularize the scientific findings: for example, the account of the mother who was forced to leave a rock concert because the child inside of her moved so much and would not calm down. Such accounts not only show the reactivity of the child to stressful situations but also seem to demonstrate that the mother can communicate with her unborn child in a special, internal, emotional dialogue. The agitation produced in the unborn child by maternal shock or panic was observed quite vividly with the use of ultrasound after an earthquake in Italy (see Ianniruberto and Tajani 1981). In several cases, the restlessness of the baby continued for up to eight hours after the shock; in some cases, this was followed by a period of markedly reduced activity that then lasted for many hours. It has also been possible using a combination of psychological test methods and ultrasound observation in experimental situations to show that maternal fear generally leads to increased activity of the child in the womb (Bergh 1990).

During the 1970s Dennis Stott (1973) carried out research into the complex long-term effects of prenatal stress. He showed that when the mother endures exceptional emotional stress before the birth in the form of a difficult personal conflict, her child usually exhibits a marked tendency to fall ill not only after birth but well into childhood. He even reported an almost one-to-one correlation. Stott surmised that prenatal emotional stress has probably such a strong effect because on a biological level it is a trigger for the termination of the pregnancy.

Benjamin Pasamanick (1966) was able to show in a series of studies carried out in the 1950s that prenatal stress

is correlated with several postnatal psychological disturbances, for example, reading difficulties, ticks, various behavior disorders, and generally reduced talent.

The neuroendocrinologist, Günter Dörner (1988) has
demonstrated that prenatal stress plays a role in the development of particular forms of male homosexuality. His
research is quite specific. The prenatal stress influences the
hormonal environment in which gender-specific brain differentiation takes place. He has conclusively demonstrated
this fact in detailed animal experiments. More recently,
Dörner has shown that more homosexuals were born in
Germany during the stressful years of the Second World War
than in the periods that immediately preceded and followed.
Furthermore, the mothers of homosexual men report having had a stressful pregnancy far more often than mothers of
heterosexual men.

It is significant for child psychotherapists and for affected parents that Lester Sontag (1966) found in his
extensive study that hyperactive and stressed babies in the
womb proved to be more fearful in childhood when confronted with aggression and were generally withdrawn and
unable to make contact with their peers. Children who had
experienced prenatal stress cried in such a peculiar way as to
give the impression that they were ill. This sort of crying can
be very penetrant, exhausting, and nerve-racking (Zeskind
1978).

The study reported by the Austrian psychologist Sepp
Schindler (1984) demonstrates the relationship between
perinatal stress and postnatal irritability in a graphic way. A
group of twenty-nine children who had experienced oxygen
deprivation during their birth were compared with children
who had not experienced any birth trauma. No difference

could be found between the two groups using development and intelligence tests. However, marked behavioral difficulties were detected in the following three categories:

1. a higher degree of sensitivity (e.g., on the day after a house-help left, a boy stayed in his room crying loudly)
2. reacting intensely and in a way not appropriate to the cause (e.g., a boy who for a long period of time vomited every day in front of his nursery)
3. increased irritability in new situations (e.g., a boy resisted getting his hair cut so much that it took three men to hold him). [p. 21]

The findings concerning the effects of prenatal stress are so disquieting that society should be encouraged to provide young parents with much better support. Nowadays parents are so financially and professionally stressed that childbearing is then an overload. The ones who carry this extra burden are usually the children themselves in their prenatal life. There are possibilities here for real social change for the better; these are crucial situations in which immediate help could be given if only our conscience could be pricked. The growing commitment of parents, midwives, gynecologists, and hospitals to the gentle birth movement is a good example of how such change can occur.

Much of the empirical evidence showing the vulnerability of the unborn child is at the same time evidence of the child's sensitivity and impressionability and especially of his or her ability to relate (Foresti 1982).

The following observation demonstrates the strong dependence of the unborn child on the mother's emotional

state. If, during ultrasound examination, a mother is told
that, when there is no spontaneous movement of her baby to
be observed on the monitor, it is evidence of a developmental disturbance, the mother naturally gets a shock when she
cannot see anything. However, this shock is always enough to
produce immediate and intense movement in her baby
(Reinold 1982).

Peter Fedor-Freybergh is one of the most significant
pioneers of prenatal psychology. Thomas Verny (Verny and
Kelly 1983) reports an anecdote of his that shows the
significance of negative feelings in a most impressive way:

> At her birth, baby Kristina was strong and healthy. . . . How-
> ever, for no apparent reason, she refused her mother's breast.
> In the baby ward, she greedily drank from a bottle. . . .
> On the next day, when she was brought to her mother, she
> refused the breast again and the same happened on the
> following days. . . . When she was put to another woman's
> breast, she immediately began searching and sucking with all
> her strength. Quite perplexed, Fedor-Freybergh talked with
> Kristina's mother. "Why does your child behave so?" he asked
> her. The mother did not know. "Were you ill during the
> pregnancy?" No, she had not been. Fedor-Freybergh then
> asked the mother bluntly: "Did you actually want the baby?"
> The woman stared up to him and answered: "No, I wanted an
> abortion but my husband wanted the child. That's why I kept
> it." That was previously unknown to Fedor-Freybergh but
> apparently not to baby Kristina. She had already painfully felt
> her mother's rejection for a long time. Then, after her birth,
> she refused to accept her mother because her mother had
> already rejected her. [p. 67]

In the past few decades, Frans Veldman (1988, 1991,
1994) has discovered that we all possess an ability to com-

municate at a deep level, a sort of spontaneous empathy, like that which unborn and small children exhibit naturally. He has named the scientific study of this sort of communication *Haptonomy*. Through "psychotactile contact"—a special sort of relating that completely embraces the other person, Veldman has demonstrated how it is possible to establish an emotional bond with the unborn child. This special bond can be objectively observed because the baby, responding to the invitation to relate, moves itself toward his hand resting on the mother's belly and snuggles up into it. Ultrasound pictures verify what is anyway clearly observable. The mother can learn this sort of empathetic contact to her child. Impartial observers have reported that babies who have experienced this prenatal, haptonomic contact develop very well after their birth and that all measurements of their development distinguish them in a dramatic way from other babies. The special significance of pre- and perinatal haptonomy can also be seen in the fact that in the mother it produces a deep relaxation and a loosening up of the pubic cartilage and the sacropelvic joint. This in turn gives the birth canal an extra 2 centimeters in width—the crucial 2 centimeters that are normally missing in human females.

Much leads us to suppose that a huge, unused, human potential lies buried in this area of prenatal relating. The infant mortality rate has been drastically reduced in the last hundred years and now there is the chance that children come to the light of day not only physically healthy but also are given all that is required for good psychological development. The specialist term for prenatal relating is *bonding* and is an essential prerequisite for postnatal bonding. The efforts to help mothers to form this prenatal bond have been intensified recently and the positive effects of emotional support around the time of birth on the health of both mother and child have been conclusively verified (Blum 1993, Klaus and Kennel 1983, Marnie 1989, Mauger 1995, Raphael-Leff 1991, Schwartz 1983, Verny and Weintraub 1992).

Conversely, to have been prenatally unwanted is quite obviously an adverse condition for future development. This was demonstrated in a detailed, longitudinal study (see Matejcek 1987) now spanning over twenty years of 220 children in the former Czechoslovakia whose mothers twice requested an abortion and were refused both times. It is certainly quite difficult to distinguish the effects of prenatal and postnatal influences. However, the offspring from un-wanted pregnancies evaluate their lives far less positively than the control group. All measures of general satisfaction with life were much lower and those of dissatisfaction much higher. Disappointment in relationships is much more fre-quent among those who were unwanted. They believe more frequently than others that "love brings more problems than pleasure." Those who were married more often reported unhappy marriage. A similar study was carried out in Sweden, which showed that juvenile criminality among unwanted children was about double that of those who had been wanted. Gerhard Amendt and Michael Schwarz (1992) have recently published a comprehensive summary of em-pirical research into the lifelong effects of having been prenatally unwanted.

An important study of the long-term effects of perinatal stress was carried out by Emmy Werner (Werner and Smith 1982). She showed among other things that the long-term consequences, even those that can be measured in adult-hood, of pre- and perinatal stress can be reduced by good postnatal care. If, however, the postnatal conditions are not good, that is, if pre- and perinatal stress comes together with early experience of family instability, then this leads to behavioral problems and difficulties in school even when all other social factors are positive.

7

Fears, Aggressions, and Fixations: Disturbances Resulting from Pre- and Perinatal Psychological Trauma

From the observations I have made as a psychotherapist, I know that the early and even the earliest experiences are not primitive, vague, reflexive, and unconscious but intense, emotional, and all-embracing. Early childhood memories have a particular fascination for many people. Whenever one succeeds in getting in touch with early impressions and memories, it is always deeply moving. Childhood experience has a very special character because the child only perceives and understands the adult world in the context of his own private feelings. A fear of the bogeyman is for the child completely real and joy at Christmas fills the whole of the child's world with a special light. From my inner experience I would like to assume that the baby before and after birth has similar and even stronger experiences than these. Perhaps our dreams and experiences in altered states of consciousness may communicate something of the intensity of these earliest impressions. I find Frans Veldman's description of early childhood awareness as "emotional consciousness" to be quite appropriate. It adequately distinguishes it from our self-reflective, adult consciousness based on language.

During our development toward adulthood, it is essential that we learn to integrate all the different layers of our experience into a harmonious whole. We can experience something of our very early feelings again through dreams, games and fantasies, bodily sensations, and emotional expectations. This is especially true for those early experiences that could not be integrated at the time of their occurrence. Experiences that could not be integrated can live on within us with a special intensity and can reveal themselves in fears and symptoms during times of temptation and stress. Here are some examples of this.

CHILDHOOD FEARS

Pre- and perinatal experiences are active in many childhood fears, which is a sign that the child has not been able to reconcile these early events with the life he leads with his parents or that something done by his parents has confused him and has reactivated a fear that he had already overcome. What on the one side seems like a disorder or a symptom is at the same time an attempt to resolve a disagreeable experience. One of the most common childhood fears is the fear of darkness, which can be triggered by various incidents.

It can mean, for example, that the child has sensed that a change in his family life is like the change that took place at his birth. As a result of this correlation, he now feels again that he is trapped in darkness, as he was during the first stages of his birth. The fear of being confined, for example of pulling tight clothes over the head, or fear of tunnels can be understood in a similar way as an unconscious repetition of fear experienced during birth.

Another very frequent fear, that of being eaten or swallowed by a wild animal, can also be understood as a reflection of the birth trauma. Fear of a very large and powerful animal can represent the fear experienced within the mother's body. Small animals are frightening perhaps because they arouse the disquieting wish to creep back into the primal security of the womb. One can guess that the small child is aware of the pre- and perinatal period of his life at the level of his emotions. A game played by a small girl is an example of this. Apparently in order to simulate the womb, she built a nest with an alarm clock in it and explained to her mother: "When I was in your tummy, it always made 'shh, shh.'" The noise made by the blood vessels, which the girl had experienced prenatally, may lie hidden behind this memory.

The child openly asks about where he came from only when this affective knowledge has been lost and there has been a move to a new level of awareness. Now the child wants to talk to his parents about his existence and identity on a more cognitive level and no longer as before in a game sequence. Otto Rank (1988) provides an example. A girl apparently is wavering between her fears of being swallowed and her first attempts to identify with her mother. Rank reports:

A little girl, 3½ years old, who was equally or even more frightened of little dogs than of big ones, was also frightened of insects (flies, bees, etc.). When the mother asked her why she was frightened of such small animals that could not do anything to her, the girl answered without any hesitation: "But they could swallow me!" Whenever she approached a little dog, she moved in the same characteristic way that an adult would when avoiding a mouse: she bent down with her legs so folded together and the knees so low that her dress practically touched the ground. It was as if she wanted to cover herself completely and prevent the animal from creeping inside. On another occasion when the mother had asked her about why she feared bees, she explained, contradicting herself, that she wanted to get inside of the bee's belly, but then not really. [p. 35]

A typical symbol for birth fear is worry about being captured by a spider, wrapped in a web, and suffocated. Similar feelings can be expressed in the image of a swamp. The very frequent fear of snakes can have its root in fear of the umbilical cord. The double symbolism of the snake, on the one hand, the bringer of health and on the other of danger, reflects the unborn child's ambivalent relationship to the umbilical cord. The English analyst Francis Mott (1964), has shown by the analysis of thousands of dreams that, as the bringer of nourishment, the umbilical cord is experienced as "healing." However, during the birth when the oxygen supply from the placenta becomes insufficient, it is experienced as dangerous and oppressive. This interpretation is supported by analogies from Egyptian mythology. The Pharaoh on his night journey, symbolizing his life in the womb, is accompanied and protected by a healing snake, whereas at dawn, a symbol of birth, he has to confront the evil snake Apophis (Hornung 1985).

To understand children's fear a little better, it is important to realize that a child's mother is first of all his uterine mother, then his birthing mother, and only then his postnatal mother in objective bodily form. This fact finds expression, for example, in the alchemist's pictures that show the early mother sitting on a whale with big, lactating breasts (Fabricius 1989). These pictures are of the nourishing postnatal mother with the uterine mother symbolized by the whale and the element of water. Another frequent symbol for the uterine mother seen in many fairy tales is the tortoise.

The fear of horses is well known from Freud's case study of the 5-year-old Little Hans. The boy's birth trauma, which was activated by seeing his mother pregnant and then the birth of a little sister, is expressed in many aspects of his phobia. In the beginning, he was only afraid in the street that a horse might bite him. That is, when he leaves the protective, maternal home, there is the danger of being bitten. This can be compared with the *vagina dentata* which he experienced as he left his protective, uterine home. The birth of the sister marks the end of his exclusive possession of the mother and a jolt to his masculine identity. At a deeper level, this activates his primal experience of his first separation from his mother. At the beginning of his phobic development, there is his fear of being left alone: the trusted mother is suddenly no longer there. In the conflict caused by his awakening masculine identity, the fearful Little Hans is reluctant to take on his new identity and to accept his penis for what it is. This would mean leaving his infantile bond to his mother behind him and, as he fears, to lose everything like at his birth. His penis becomes the umbilical cord that maintains his bond to his mother but that is in a fatal way also threatened by birth and cutting. Freud was aware of the maternal aspects of the boy's problem. However, he tried to explain it only in the context of the father. For Freud, the predominant childhood feelings were fear and protection of the father.

Another example of childhood anxiety that has become famous because Freud reported it is the case of the Wolfman. The Wolfman dreamed, between the ages of 3 and 5, how, as he lay in bed, the window would open. Then he was frightened that he would be eaten by wolves that were sitting in a tree. It is also possible to understand this dream in the context of a birth trauma. It is also the case that the Wolfman as small child was in conflict with his developing masculinity. His perinatal experience was reawakened by the fact that he had to free himself from his infantile dependence on the mother. The dream is to be understood in the following way: when the window opens, the room, which symbolizes the all-embracing, uterine mother, turns into the "devouring birth-mother" symbolized by the wolves. According to Dowling, we can understand the tree, which at first appears not to be troublesome as a projection of the placenta, that is, as a symbol of the prenatal mother. The other symbols in the boy's dream, the winter landscape and the tree that appeared to have broken trunk, treetop, and branches, indicate that the Wolfman had also suffered a prenatal trauma.

CHILDHOOD MISTAKES

Children in situations of conflict can fall back into previous patterns of behavior where they may feel more secure. The child who can already walk begins again to crawl, the child who had already been weaned wants to be back at the breast, and so on. These regressive tendencies can go back even beyond babyhood into the womb. A typical example is that of a patient whose lips had played with a damp cloth directly after her difficult birth and who then could not be separated from her "cuddly cloth" during her whole childhood. She was trying to find feelings of prenatal reassurance again after her birth.

Thumb-sucking can be a revival of breast-sucking but just as easily of sucking on the umbilical cord or of the thumb before birth. Similarly, wetting and messing the bed can signify a regression to babyhood or a flight even further back into the womb where there were no such cares. The deep fear that many children have of losing their parents and their general separation anxiety can have roots in a real, abrupt separation or in a difficult birth that the child was not helped to overcome.

NEUROTIC SYMPTOMS

As early as 1924, Otto Rank stated with impressive lucidity: "Analysis has proven that fear lies at the heart of every neurotic disorder. And because we have recognised through Freud that primal fear comes from the birth trauma, the relationship to it must in fact be open to proof everywhere, just as it is in the case of the child's emotional reactions" (p. 63).

However, Rank underestimated the difficulty of realizing the content of his statement—the amount of confrontation and transcendence of one's own repression and the expansion of consciousness that is necessary here.

It took several more years until the Hungarian psychoanalyst Nandor Fodor (1949) was able to take the next step and realize the full significance of prenatal trauma. However, this knowledge has only reached a broader public thanks to the use of LSD, hypnosis, and primal therapy, all of which have helped to overcome the repression of birth memories. Perhaps, however, a general change in attitudes has also been important. People do not so often nowadays seek security in an idealized leader or utopian state but understand the new, cultural ideal of democratic responsibility. To demonstrate Rank's basic principle that every neurotic symptom has a perinatal root, it is only possible here to give a few examples. The generality of this theory and also its boundaries have not been adequately tested as yet.

From observations made in psychotherapeutic practice, it is clear that changes in life can arouse neurotic fears and complaints. This is so because change always touches our primal experience of transition that occurred at our birth. Put another way, change reminds the unconscious mind of our very first fearful, separation from our mother. One can also say that we look at life in the light of our earliest, emotional experiences. When these primal experiences cannot be integrated within later psychological development, elements of the birth, for example, can show themselves in neurotic symptoms. Put bluntly, neurotic symptoms speak in a perinatal dialect.

Phobias provide particularly impressive examples of fear connected with the events of birth. Our unconscious can imagine a paternoster (elevator) to be a threatening birth movement, or a tunnel becomes the oppressive birth canal. Such emotional reactions occur with the same totality as in early childhood and the sufferer can only hope to avoid the things that trigger the deep regression. Very often the simple explanation that the phobia is connected with birth can bring relief.

Anxiety depression can have roots in the first phase of birth, the opening of the cervix. A depressive patient, for example, could not get rid of the threatening idea that everything was heading toward an all-engulfing chasm. He had experienced a very difficult and prolonged birth. His mother had never accepted her femininity and fought vehemently against the processes of birth. The mother and the child were left alone in this terrible situation. This corresponded exactly to the patient's feelings toward life. The trauma was actually reactivated when, in tragic circumstances, the man lost the partner with whom he had planned to spend the rest of his life. The marriage itself had been a sort of flight back into the security of the womb. The death of the partner had meant the dissolution of this fantasy and the reactivation of feelings of being born.

The pattern of symptoms found in obsessional neuroses very commonly also reflects a preoccupation with birth. Usually it is a case of a complex interplay of pre-, peri-, and postnatal stress. The child who was already damaged and frightened in the womb is unable to cooperate with the mother during the birth and often has to put up with obsessional behavior in the family afterward. The child never gets to experience real care and as a result his attitude to life is built on painful experiences, themselves determined as if by magic by obsessional rituals. Ritual washing is an attempt to restore prenatal purity and reverse the experience of birth.

A patient, for example, has developed a complicated system of obsessions that were intended to preserve the fiction that she never ever touched the ground, in fact that she had not even been born. When involuntary contact did occur, it was redressed by ritual washing. I have often heard patients express the spontaneous idea that their own actions and movements were the cause of their perinatal calamity. The aforementioned patient feared that she could cause a world catastrophe by particular blunders or when she picked up the telephone. Numerous ceremonies of opening and shutting a door were attempts to restore her state of life in the womb.

The apparent ease with which associations have been made in the examples above between adult experience and pre- and perinatal events may seem strange. Perhaps the consideration of metaphors that are directly related to the experience of birth may offer a key to understanding here. Such phrases are often connected with an individual's birth experience in a striking manner. Good examples of such expressions are "there is no way out" from someone who had a prolonged delivery or the phrase "I feel torn in all directions" from someone where the use of forceps was necessary during the birth. The American psychologist Sandra Landsman (1989) has collected many examples: "Banging one's head against a wall," "There is no solution," "I feel drugged," "There is nobody to help me," "I must always do everything alone," "I never succeed" (pp. 33ff). These examples already begin to demonstrate that one's whole attitude to life can be seriously affected by pre- and perinatal events. The psychoanalyst Alfred Adler had already discovered as early as 1907 that a person can be disturbed by prenatal experiences in a way leading to inferiority complexes. Adler at first thought more of maternal illness or traumas caused by poison. Nowadays, as a result of the studies carried out by Stott and Kafkalides, for example, we know that emotional rejection of the pregnancy, maternal conflict, and fear are very important factors. I had a patient who suffered from terrible attacks of unworthiness and helplessness in situations of stress. Further analysis revealed that there had been an attempted abortion in the middle of the pregnancy. Many examples of cases similar to this can be found in the book *Ungewollte Kinder* (*Unwanted Children*), edited by Helga Häsing and me (1994). The Greek psychiatrist Kafkalides (1995) closes a report concerning the LSD-treatment of a 26-year-old woman with the following words:

> In a later consultation, a patient made the following comment about her feelings towards life: "My everyday feeling of being despised and ridiculed, of being a nobody, unable to make contact, of being a woman—all of that is based upon the rejection and rebuff which I experienced in the womb. I see my womb experience as a threatening monster and see it in the people around me who actually reject me just like the womb did. As a fetus in the womb, I felt my mother's rejection as an attempt to kill me. . . . Actually I am still living in the womb. [p. 46]

THE PSYCHOLOGICAL EFFECTS OF PRENATAL STRESS ON CHILDREN AND ADULTS

Even though only a few psychotherapists are aware of the prenatal roots of neurotic symptoms, so many observations have now been made that they can be categorized. The English theologian and psychotherapist Frank Lake (1979) produced such a scheme as early as the 1970s. He considers the mother's negative relationship to her unborn child as the cause of so-called distress syndrome. The child's relationship to the mother is expressed by the way in which the placenta is experienced. One piece of evidence for this hypothesis is that the symbol of the Tree of Life plays a central role in all cosmologies. This tree can be understood as a projection of the placenta, which we experienced before our birth (see Dowling 1987a). The tree is a sort of embodiment of the maternal being upon which everything depends. When the unborn child experiences emotional stress it is important that it copes with its immense feelings by splitting, projective displacement, and a recurring, defensive posture. The patterns of these coping mechanisms can be reconstructed by comparing the results of research using LSD with the psychodynamic inferences obtained from observations of psychological symptoms. According to Lake, (1979) the main defensive reactions are the following:

- Hysterical splitting, by which negative emotion is collected within the body in the vicinity of the navel: The body's insides are bad and dangerous, whereas everything outside is held to be good. I am reminded of one of my patients who was born after a pregnancy full of ambivalence and rejection. She had the feeling that the whole of her lower body was full of dirt and filth. She suffered from the strongest feelings of insecurity but seemed on the surface to be happy and content. The internal erosion of her self-esteem made it impossible for her to develop a feminine identity.
- Phobic projection, in which the negative emotion is experienced as a threat coming from without: The placenta is threatening and is later symbolized by spiders and squids. The threat posed by the umbilical cord appears later in the fear of snakes. Good objects are also found outside. As Lake comments, birth complications are often to be found behind claustrophobia. Phobic reactions are very common and can be very resistant to therapy. The patients are in

permanent flight from phobic objects, search for security in a protective person, and are always building new havens of retreat.

- Anxiety-depressive ambivalent reaction, which appears when good and evil influences occur together: The unborn child tries to defend and then becomes tense. He wants to get rid of the umbilical cord, which of course would mean his death. He feels trapped in rage. Many patients who live in destructive conditions of dependence show this reaction. Every attempt to become independent is threatened with punishment.

- Obsessional neurotic dissociation, whereby evil is placed inside and outside: The person feels unable to control the influx of disgusting and offensive emotions. There is a deep fear of touching the umbilical cord. Rituals of detachment set in. I had a patient who had had to withstand a pregnancy during which the mother had been very ill, had been badly undernourished, and had had strong feelings of rejection towards the child. In her puberty, the patient had begun to make bizarre rubbing movements in a bus—the bus having obvious womb significance. This ritual developed into evermore far-ranging obsessions.

Other defense reactions to extreme levels of negative affect are the paranoid defense—the construction of a persecutory world—and the schizoid defense—the avoidance of all close contact and withdrawal into a private, inner world.

These suggestions are first attempts to gain orientation in an area of life still in need of much research. However, I have presented them here so that the beginnings of a prenatal psychological theory of the neuroses can become clear. When massive, prenatal trauma has occurred and there has been no chance for restitution in childhood, then the impulsive affects can inundate later experience. Only long-term therapy offers any promise here (Costa Segui 1995, Dowling 1992, 1994, Findeisen 1992, Galati 1996, Ingalls 1996, Noble 1993, Wasdell 1994).

It has remained until now little known that the relationship between partners provides a very common setting for the staging of primal emotions. They can be relived here in unchanging repetition. As is the case with the treatment of phobias, the simple hint that there is a connection to birth and prenatal existence can bring considerable relief. On the other hand, the prenatal roots of relationship disorders also explains why intense partner conflicts are very difficult to influence and resolve. The conflict is fueled by the early trauma (Dowling 1994).

PSYCHOSOMATIC ILLNESS

It is possible to begin to distinguish between psychosomatic symptoms that are rooted in prenatal disturbances and those that are perinatally determined. The latter, the perinatal symptoms, are easier to understand on the simple grounds that birth is a drastic and visible event. It was these that were first discovered and described by Otto Rank (1988):

> Direct reproductions of the birth trauma can be produced by . . . all neurotic breathing disorders (asthma) which revive the experience of suffocation, headache (migraine) which can be used in so many ways and which goes back to

the especially painful involvement of the head during the birth and finally and very directly fits which incidentally one can already observe in very small children, even newborns, as further attempts to deal with the original birth trauma. [p. 67]

This introduces the field of prenatal psychosomatics. Even when one tries to imagine the birth process, this can stimulate feelings that can lead to a deeper insight into the following summary of symptoms produced by Arthur Janov (1984). He made the following list from many case studies: feelings of being strangled, chronic tiredness, localized pain, numbness, pressure, feelings of annihilation, breathlessness, tension in neck and shoulders, feelings of being squashed, chronic physical tension, generalized pain, habitual head and neck posture, impulsiveness, dizziness, asthma, headache and migraine, pain in the joints, and bronchitis.

Two examples from Janov's work can serve here to illustrate these statements. One patient had a pathological head and neck posture:

"After several weeks of birth primalling in which I re-experienced extraordinarily strong pain in the back of my head and in my shoulders, I began to feel an incredible resolution of all the physical tensions which had been frozen into these parts my whole life long. The muscles and sinews around my neck seemed to be miraculously freed from a life-long constriction." [p. 182]

Another of Janov's patients who suffered from pains in his face wrote:

"During my birth primals, I always felt a lot of pain in my face. I also feel pain there when I sleep. I feel as if the right side is being pushed out. I asked my mother about my birth and she said that the delivery came to a complete standstill after which I came out with a 'visibly squashed face, especially above the nose.' That fits to what I have always felt in my face—what I must have felt in the birth canal as the complication occurred. My face was squashed and I felt danger." [p. 182]

Because established psychological research has avoided questions about the reactivation of early traumas in psychosomatic symptoms, only a few empirical studies have been carried out. Lee Salk (1974), for example, studied asthma. He is also the author of the well-known work (1973) about postnatal recall of the mother's heartbeat as heard in the womb. He compared the birth reports of thirty asthmatic children with those of a control group. The results were astonishingly significant. The asthma group had experienced far more perinatal complications, so that this correlation can be taken as suggested. This corresponds to the experience I have had as a psychotherapist. One patient had frequent dreams of suffocation and drowning. In many dreams, he was drifting in a canal and he had to try to stay above water by swimming or he would drown. His first dream during the therapy concerned a shaft. He climbed out of it with the help of the therapist who provided him with a ladder. This is a very graphic representation of the process of getting free from his perinatal predicament. During his childhood and youth, this problem had been confounded with a complicated dependency problem by the mother. The asthma had developed out of the feeling that he was being crushed and suffocated in his marriage. The asthma attacks were also triggered by a feeling of suffocation.

In the case of another asthma patient, unlike the

previous one, the circumstances of his birth were known in detail. The mother had tried to start the birth by jumping from a stool. As a result, the birth was at first forced and then delayed. In situations of stress, the patient always felt the danger that had accompanied his birth. Everything then depended on getting through or not getting through. In his imagination, the journey to work became a struggle to get through the birth canal with dreadful delays. He had to drive very skillfully in order nevertheless to get there in time.

The connections to birth can be very obvious in cases of headache. It is always the case that the perinatal conflict has been reinforced in a complicated way by later problems and that the reactivation of the perinatal sensations expresses the other difficulties as well. In the case of one patient, a journey through a glen and the accompanying feeling of being hemmed in was enough, when he was tense, to trigger depression and headache. The analysis itself was regularly concerned with agonizing impasse, with locked doors, with feelings of not getting through. Finally, in several sessions, elements of the traumatic birth were reproduced and to a large extent overcome.

It was the ambivalence between suffering in front of a locked door and the fear of being destroyed in the birth trauma that pulled the patient this way and that. His situation after birth was determined by the fact that, because there were several older children, he felt that there was no place for him in the family; even here, he could not get through and achieve a recognized autonomy.

The perinatal connection is often very apparent in the experience of patients who suffer epilepsy (Ferenczi 1964b, Schilder 1973). Indeed, this was discovered early in psycho-analysis. The patients report again and again that the attacks are connected with the fear of being annihilated and the feeling of not getting through. The author Sue Cooke (see Rausch 1988a) describes her attacks as follows: "Only we know why we hit ourselves. It happens with me because I have been buried in a grave or underwater in a deep, black ocean and in panic I am trying to get out of the depths into light again. Every muscle of my body is involved in this enormous effort, in this struggle to survive" (p. 133).

It must also be remembered here that the birth trauma and the memory of it can only have a long-term effect when it was not possible during childhood and youth—because of, for example, conflict in the parental relationship—for the individual to resolve the perinatal threat in various positive interactions.

As far as I know, the perinatal roots of the so-called heart neurosis have not been examined. This neurosis appears in situations of separation and consists of a deadly fear that the heart will stop. The attack of fear must also here be understood in the context of a postnatal conflict between dependency and detachment. Because of the fear that a partner might leave them or they might lose their profession, the patients enter relationships of dependence and try to maintain the earliest form of security. When this dependence is called into question and a separation and a step toward maturity becomes necessary, the original separation anxiety and fear of developmental change that occurred at their birth is reactivated. Very often it is a bereavement that makes a person aware of the uncertainty of all bonds and triggers the heart neurosis. I understand the symptom itself to be a repetition of the terrifying shock that can accompany the changeover in circulation during a difficult birth. I am fairly convinced that this changeover can be a frightening shock to the circulatory system when the umbilical cord is cut too soon and too abruptly. The organism is then forced to perform a transformation that should take minutes in the space of a few seconds. As a result of perinatal trauma, the world inside of the mother, the magical-hypnotic, prenatal bond to the mother, cannot be properly differentiated from the external world and the postnatal relationship to the mother. They remain bound to one another.

When patients as a result of external stress fall back or regress to a birth fixation for the first time, the original separation anxiety fills their whole life. Leaving their house or their car, both of which can symbolize the womb, can trigger awful panic. The unresolved developmental conflict is lived on in such scenes symbolic of birth. The positive significance of such symptoms can be seen in the fact that the steps toward maturity that have become necessary for the individual presuppose that they at last experience and begin to come to terms with some of their birth fears.

While perinatal damage is itself patterned according to the birth process and is therefore easier to recognize, prenatal trauma is often difficult to distinguish; it is, nevertheless, determined by prenatal conditions. This can be clearer within indirect injuries, for example, as in the case of attempted abortion. A fetus that has suffered this can in later life experience sudden attacks of weakness and unconsciousness or paranoia. Difficult disorders of the vegetative nervous system with muscle tension can be the expression of continuous fetal stress. I had a patient who came for psychotherapy seeking euthanasia. To die was her only wish. She was tormented by diffuse pain and feelings of despair and had various psychosomatic symptoms. She appeared to me to be nothing other than a bundle of negativity. It was possible for me to contact her mother about my suspicion of a prenatal trauma. The pregnancy had been stressful because the mother had been in desperate circumstances and basically she had wanted to get rid of the child. This fact had never been discussed. The mother had tried to hide everything within herself and to appear to the child to be carefree. As a result, the child had not been able to find any outlet for the latent sadness that she felt. She was only allowed to exist as her mother's "sunshine." The patient's life was so terrible because—just as during her prenatal existence burdened by her mother's unhappiness—there was no place of rest for her in this world. Even lying in the sunshine in a meadow triggered unbearable pain and the feeling that she was burning. It was not possible for this patient to give any form to her negative tensions. Even under minimal stress, it is quite possible that the negative affect coming from the mother will be organized by the fetus into a particular pattern of pain and tension, for example, in the digestive tract, in the back muscles, or in the skin. Then it is a case of what psychosomatic medicine describes as a deep distortion and distress rooted in conflict of the whole organism.

It is sometimes less complicated to find a connection between dermatologic illnesses and prenatal experience. One patient who had been exposed to strong rejection during the pregnancy and had developed neurodermatitis after birth dreamt again and again of collapsing houses and buildings that then began to burn. Because he had been given away after his birth, in later meetings with his mother even the slightest conflict was always liable to cause a rapid return to the level of the prenatal ambivalence. The full skin complaint could appear in minutes when, for example, he met his mother during the holidays and did not know for sure if she was going to leave him again after a short time. However, this patient was able in therapy to reestablish contact with good prenatal states and in his dreams and relationships activate desires for and feelings of prenatal, symbiotic union. This occurred hand in hand with a disappearance of his symptoms. In situations where this desire for union broke down, the disorder reappeared.

The case of one young patient shows just how easy it can be to experience fetal sensations. This 13-year-old gave up learning to swim because of damage to her ears, although there was actually no real danger. However, even swimming was enough to activate a regression to the fetal state and she thereby lost all orientation. Just as a fetus paddles free in its primal sea and may lose its sense of balance under stress, so she began swimming toward the bottom or straight ahead or to the side. A similar loss of balance occurred in a patient as soon as she was in darkness. She would begin to totter, perhaps just like the fetus does when it loses clear contact with the mother. The explanation of these severe afflictions, by suggesting their connection to prenatal experiences, can be very relieving because such weaknesses can themselves be very annoying and discouraging.

DEVIANT DEVELOPMENT AND CRIMINALITY

It is known that asocial development often occurs when very early fears and aggressions caused by pre- and perinatal trauma or by "intrauterine hospitalism" (Hau 1982) cannot be sorted out because of adverse postnatal conditions. They are then continually enacted and often with little disguise or transformation into symbols. The classic example is the Oedipus saga where the aggression suffered pre- and perinatally is later lived out in the murder of the father and the tendency to regress to the womb in incest with the mother. The immediacy and intensity of early fears is the cause of the great difficulty they pose for therapists. Here is a dream from a juvenile delinquent in which a whole series of pre- and perinatal trauma reveals itself:

"I am driving along a street together with my grandmother in her car. Suddenly the street in front of us opens and we are in a huge cave, in a sort of cooking pot. The street winds its way high up the walls and then crisscross through the cave. To the right and left of the street there are doors. When they open for a short time, we can see a huge fire and the Devil who is torturing people. We are terribly frightened because an attack can come suddenly from all sides" [Rauchfleisch 1987, p. 144]

The connections between prenatal stress and later criminality have been dramatically illustrated in the conversation protocols published by Balthasar Gareis and Eugen Wiesnet (1974):

"When I was in the third month of the pregnancy with Anton, I wanted to get married. When my father found out—I was seventeen at the time—he became absolutely furious and beat me. I could not get married because the man was unacceptable to my father. . . . From the moment he knew I was pregnant, I did not have another quiet moment. When I came home late in the evening and he realized that I had been with Anton's father, I was unable to sleep the whole night long because he had abused and beaten me so much. I would cry the whole night. I even tried to take my life at that time but I did not find the courage to do it because I remembered my child. . . . In the time before the birth, I became so nervous that I would begin to cry over the smallest thing. . . . Finally, it got to the point that even Anton's father didn't like me anymore because I let myself get so rundown. . . . Anton's birth was the worst experience of my life. After his birth, his left arm was paralysed. . . . When I was breast-feeding him, I cried all the time so that Anton began to cry as well. Anton was often ill. He was restless, nervous and very easily frightened. . . . My other two children are completely different. But during the pregnancies with them, there weren't any unpleasant events. Nowadays I think that the pregnancy is the most important time in the life of a child. Anton has a good heart. He didn't want to murder. It is not his fault that he is the way he is." [p. 16]

As a boy, Anton had occasionally attracted attention in school because of his diffident attitude, irritability and his unpredictable behavior, everything from self-mutilation to massive aggression.

When he was seventeen, Anton brutally murdered a sixteen-year-old girl. He killed her most cruelly by multiple strangulation, choking her for a few minutes at a time. Anton committed the crime without any emotional excitement. . . . His personality disturbance can be seen in heightened irritability, tendency to mistrust and jealousy. In addition, he has moods which can rise to exhibitions of suicide. Anton reacts in a peculiar way to unusual stress and opposition in his surroundings. On the one hand, he shows the tendency to get his way at any price and on the other he avoids difficulties, is undecided and becomes sentimental." [p. 15]

Here is a second report about a 16-year-old youth called Uwe who committed robbery with grievous injury to the victim. The mother's statement:

"Actually it all began in the pregnancy. After I realised that I was pregnant with him, I went to the doctor's and just couldn't believe that I was going to have another child. My husband was also so disappointed because we only had a small apartment. You just wouldn't believe how unhappy I was about the pregnancy. I was so nervous and at the end of my tether. I was sometimes dreadfully unhappy and felt such anger towards the baby. Sometimes I even thought about abortion but that would have been so unjust. I was so nervous at that time that it showed in my face. I actually got a twitch which stayed for quite a while. Even today, when I get nervous, as, for example, when I heard about the crime, the twitch starts up again. The agitation must have had an effect on the child. He was very weak after his birth and nearly died. That's when I felt a deep pity and looked at things differently. Then he could not tolerate my milk, drank badly and most of the time vomited everything out again. As a result he hardly put on weight and was often ill. He permanently had fever, sore throat and pimples. I just don't know where that came from. He was so nervous and restless that he stayed well behind in his development. . . . You can still notice to this day that he is unquiet and uneasy. . . . When he is nowadays agitated, then his eye always twitches. He always gets into a rage so quickly. Both of these he got from me during the pregnancy. The other three children are completely different. . . . But despite everything, Uwe isn't to blame. If only I hadn't got so upset when I found out that he was on his way." [p. 18]

I imagine that some crimes are in a way the living out of prenatal suffering and agony, as if the hellish dream described above were put into practice. This always presupposes that the pre- and perinatal trauma could not be cleared up in the time after birth. In Germany, the now

famous case of Jürgen Barsch who murdered children in a
cave bears the traces of the reactivation of an abortion
trauma, a prenatal experience that is deflected onto the
victim through sexual perversion. Barsch reported that he
used to hallucinate a crime many times before he carried it
out (see Föster 1984). The information about the beginning
of his life is sparse but does not exclude the possibility of all
sorts of negative experiences. He was born outside of
marriage: "He remained in a clinic during his first year of
life. His mother, who in any case did not want to have him,
died shortly after his birth" (p. 21).

The results of statistical research into the relationship of
juvenile criminality and pre- and perinatal experience are
impressive. The following figures are taken from Gareis and
Wiesnet (1974): "Sixty-seven percent of juvenile prisoners
come from a broken home. Only 32% were born within
marriage. In 57% of the cases, the baby was unwanted and in
33% the mother was unhappy and psychologically stressed"
(p. 112). The authors comment, "The child experiences
from the very beginning of his life the basic feeling of being
unwanted. . . . Very often, later in the course of arguments
in the family, the youth is reminded that he had been
unwanted" (p. 113).

As an example of this, here is the statement of a
17-year-old young woman with a criminal history: "At the
time of my birth, my parents were not married. It was then
a forced marriage because of what people would say. As a
result, my parents have never really liked me. I have always
felt that I was rejected even from birth onwards. I often
remember life at home with horror" (p. 117).

One can also see a reenactment of pre- and perinatal
trauma in the way in which society deals with its deviant
members. This is especially so in the case of punishments

carried out in the Middle Ages. They can easily be deciphered as pre- and perinatal injuries. Crime itself is a failed attempt to discover one's true identity. It fails precisely because of the fixation caused by the early trauma. The situation, however, becomes much more complicated because society, in order to gain some relief from its own pre- and perinatal fears, acts them out upon its deviants. Progress in our systems of criminal justice does reflect, albeit in a limited way, an increase in awareness. Primitive projection and reenactment of our deepest fears has been restricted.

SUICIDE

On the basis of empirical investigation, the way in which a person commits suicide follows the pattern of his or her birth (Jacobson 1988). When the birth was connected with forceful intervention, then death is achieved by force, for example, throwing oneself in front of a train or shooting. When the birth took place with the use of narcosis, the death is attempted by means that lead to unconsciousness, for example, sleeping pills.

Studies have emphasized that the person who attempts suicide wishes to be united again in a primitive way with the mother. This seems to be possible only by a reversal of birth and a return to life in the womb. In this respect, suicide represents a distorted attempt at reunion or rebirth, an attempt to rebuild a hopeless life. The hopelessness itself can also have a root in a pre- and perinatal damage. The person actually seeks a new resolution of the danger that at the time he could not come to terms with. He is trying to start his life afresh. The study that the psychiatrist David Rosen (1975) carried out of people who had survived jumping from the Golden Gate Bridge in San Francisco supports this view. After they had gone through this awful experience, they had all managed to start a new life. The fateful dive was for all of them a way of disposing of a primitive fear of death and had opened for them the chance of starting all over again.

Sadly, however, all too often regularly repeated suicide attempts do not bring about a new beginning but rather imprison the person in the original trauma. The original stress or difficulty is just too big to be sorted out in the present. Here is an example of this from Eva Eichenberger (1987), a psychotherapist living in Bern:

> Mrs. A. is a young, artistically talented woman who at first appearances makes a really lively and fearless impression. However, it is the case that she has reacted to every demand that has ever been placed upon her with panic and depression. She was unable to practise her profession as teacher, she is separated from her husband, she is only able to do a limited amount of work, is disoriented and frightened. One of the phrases which she repeated again and again during our first meeting was: "I will never succeed!", the other, "I'll kill myself!" Even in the introductory conversation, she saw her obsession with suicide as going back to the fact that she was the sixth out of seven children, that she had endangered her mother's life during the birth and that her existence was to blame for her father's financial worries. . . .
>
> The family had seven children, the last three being conceived against the doctor's advice. Their births had been so dangerous as to endanger not only the life of the mother but also that of the baby. The mother had been sure that she would not survive Mrs. A's birth. In the event, she had proved to be smaller than the previous three babies. The mother, however, contracted a severe uterine infection. She became

so weak that she was frightened to go to sleep because she feared she would then die. Mrs. A. was given into the care of others who were very happy to look after her. It is said that the mother didn't ask after her baby for weeks. Mrs. A. reported that she could easily imagine her mother's exhaustion and depression. She had herself gone through "similar states" when she had got into situations where she was under too much stress and as a result had become ill. During her childhood and puberty, Mrs. A. had never felt that she was a real individual. . . .

As Mrs. A. tried with me to feel her way back into the state of the unborn and newborn child that she had once been, she soon recognised that her suicidal tendencies and her fear that even the simple demands of everyday life could overwhelm her were old feelings. Her tendency to regress, that is, her defensive attitude towards life, is so very powerful because her mother had expected that she and her baby would die during the birth. Then she had been exhausted and secretly loathed her baby. She had thus been given hardly any support and encouragement to live. [p. 151]

It is my impression that patients with chronic suicidal tendencies can only be helped when the life-threatening events that occurred at the very earliest stages of their existence are taken into account. The significance of these experiences cannot be underestimated. Puberty triggers a greater danger of suicide because during this phase of development the person must leave the world of childhood and make the transition to adulthood. Exactly this transition can reactivate the experience of birth and the individual can be overwhelmed by the same feelings and sensations that occurred during the transition to postnatal life. Anyone who has ever seen just how exhausted, blue, and shocked some babies are after their birth can imagine how dreadful it is when a person relives such feelings. This is especially frightening for those who were exposed to prenatal stress. The child is already damaged even before it goes through birth. This was the case for one of my patients. He relived various primal sensations during crises or situations of stress with his parents. In particular, he felt that his arms and legs were lifeless and dead, as if the blood had literally stood still in his veins. To find some sort of a solution, he had to slit his arms open. This brought him some relief. Cutting the arms is a relatively frequent method of committing suicide during puberty. Terence Dowling understands these strange feelings in the arms and legs to have their origin in the changes of the baby's circulation that can occur during birth. Circulatory collapse before birth, narcosis during the birth, and the alterations that must take place in the baby's circulation after birth can all be associated with such awful feelings.

Because suicide is such a dramatic and specific event, it is easy to carry out statistical studies. As a result of his LSD research, Grof guessed that aggressive methods of suicide are related to the second and third perinatal matrix (the phases of uterine contractions and expulsion of the child), while suicide brought about by drugs is connected to the use of anesthetics during birth. These assumptions have now been statistically verified in the work of Bertil Jacobson (1988). His study was inspired by epidemiological research that had been carried out in the United States. This research showed that the form of suicide depends on the year of birth. The pattern of each year is constant and independent of whether the person born in that year committed suicide at the age of 20, 40, or 60. However, the pattern for those born between 1920 and 1925 is different from the pattern for those born between 1925 and 1930 (Hellon 1980, Murphy and Wetzel 1980).

The results of this study have shown that birth complications exercise considerable influence on the method of
suicide. It is now assumed that the alteration in the suicide
pattern for each year reflects the changes that occur in the
conditions of birth. These conditions change in a noticeable
way as a result, for example, of scientific and medical
innovations. The study carried out in Sweden as a control
confirmed this hypothesis. As a part of this study, hospitals in
Stockholm that had different obstetric practices were compared with one another. A different pattern of suicide was
found among the adults born in each of the various hospitals, each performing a different sort of delivery. The studies
just mentioned also encouraged Lee Salk (1985) to carry out
a statistical study of adolescent suicide. Epidemiological
studies have shown that the suicide rate among adolescents
has risen continuously in the last decades. This could be
partly understood as a result of the developments in obstetrics and the improvements that have taken place in neonatal
medicine. Many more children who not so long ago would
most surely have died now survive extremely traumatic birth
complications. When these traumatized children enter puberty and face the stress of further development, they have a
higher risk of suicide. Salk compared the birth report of
fifty-two adolescents who had committed suicide with two
control groups, and the statistical correlation was astonishing. The suicide group had experienced far more birth
complications than members of the control groups. Especially noticeable differences were found in three categories:
"prolonged asphyxia, chronic maternal illness during the
pregnancy and no medical investigation of the pregnancy
within the first twenty weeks" (p. 626). This demonstrates
that not only perinatal but also prenatal distress has a
significant influence on a person's tendency toward suicide.

PSYCHOSIS

A new study carried out by the child psychiatrist Reinhart Lempp (1984) has led to the formulation of a developmental-psychological model of the causes of schizophrenia. Schizophrenia is described as a disorder of a person's relationship to reality. The symptoms are confused processes of regression toward the center of the disturbance. Alongside various postnatal factors, pre- and perinatal traumas are also specified as causes. Numerous studies of the factors causing or promoting the later development of schizophrenia have provided evidence of the significance of pre- and perinatal injuries. Research in prenatal psychology can demonstrate that this disordered relationship to reality begins in the prenatal phase of life. This research, which is based primarily on individual cases, has partly achieved the status of an empirical study. A statistical analysis of the fantasies of patients who had become schizophrenic during puberty established that they contained reliable information about events that had occurred at the time of birth (Telerent et al. 1991). This is supported by many single observations of the reappearance of pre- and perinatal experiences in psychotic individuals. Ultimately, one can say that a person has become psychotic when he or she shows pre- and perinatal patterns of reaction to stress, that is, begins to act again as he or she did in the pre- and perinatal phase of life.

Pre- and perinatal influences are seen in the feelings that a psychotic person has about himself, that he feels himself to be unreal and in danger of disintegrating inside. The physical effects are equally clear. The psychotic person's basic attitude to life is determined by panic and overwhelming fear. The world seems to be a dungeon from which there is no way out. It is easy to interpret this as being arrested in a negative prenatal state.

A nihilistic attitude to one's self is characteristic of this. Here are some examples of this threatened identity taken from the therapeutic work of an American psychiatrist, Moira Pyle Fitzpatrick (1988). A young schizophrenic describes her private experience during a psychotic episode: "I am in a trap, enclosed in a milky, white fog. I push out as hard as I can. I am out of breath, I cannot get any air. I thrash around, I roll from side to side, I try to hurt, I am beside myself with rage. A dark hole with a glimmer of light is pursuing me. Inside, I collapse. I feel strangled, I cannot breathe, I become engulfed in darkness" (p. 264). Another young patient says: "Hands are pursuing me, they want to kill me."

Another of Fitzpatrick's schizophrenic patients had had to face her mother's existential conflict and fundamental rejection in her prenatal life. Her mother had also become paralyzed during the pregnancy and was not allowed to take any medication. She later blamed her daughter for the paralysis, which remained. The patient described her experience during the therapeutic regression:

"The pain, the unbelievable pain, the feeling that all my vital energies were being taken away from me, my physical energy, the air for me to breathe, everything was taken from me. My mother's body wrapped itself around me and wanted to squash me. And I remember how I turned this way and that in order to escape, in order not to be squashed and how I was fighting at the same time for my life. Every support for my life had been cut away from me. . . . I felt that my mother wanted to starve me out and to suck the life out of me through the umbilical cord. It was more like she was taking my life away than that she was giving it to me." [p. 264]

A fundamental aspect of schizophrenic experience is the feeling of not having been wanted, of not having attained real existence. The most fundamental support before birth was missing and with it the energy to cope with life in the postnatal world. These are also the central themes mentioned by the Swiss psychiatrist and psychoanalyst Gaetano Benedetti (1983) in the summary of his experience with schizophrenics in therapy. He speaks of schizophrenia as a negative existence, a negative identity, of the schizophrenic's self-hatred and relationship to the world as one of mutual negation. Many schizophrenics believe that they are bad and trash, and were starved, terrorized, and poisoned in the womb. In insanity, prenatal crises often show themselves without any disguise whatsoever in such dramatic depictions as these. The patient can also be quite clearly aware without the mediation of any symbolism of the prenatal associations. One of Fitzpatrick's patients said: "I feel in-utero, inside, not outside. If you're a fetus, you know it. There is nothing you can do" (p. 264). The process of birth can also be quite explicitly expressed in insanity. Another of Fitzpatrick's patients described how her birth began with terrific pressure on her head. She had the feeling that she had had to defend herself against her mother's and the doctor's manipulations:

"They do not have the right to force me to go through this agony of coming out in such darkness. I say no!" Afterward there was a transformation in this patient's experience and she got herself into an incredible rage and felt how she was falling into a tunnel. Her breathing became panicky and she felt threatened from every side. The image of a black panther came up and then she felt that her body was disintegrating. Her life was threatened. Finally she went along with events and felt she had been born. [p. 264]

The extreme prenatal stress that one hears in these reports and from questioning of mothers may also influence the development of the brain, in particular that of the limbic system, the cerebral center of emotions. Results from this report thus do not support the idea that schizophrenia is inherited. Prenatal stress also causes extreme hormonal imbalance, which in turn influences brain differentiation.

One can muse whether an unconscious premonition about the prenatal roots of psychosis lies hidden in the theory that psychoses are endogenous, that is, they come from "inside." In that case, the schizophrenics' so-called threshold handicap, as described by the psychiatrist Klaus Conrad (1966), would reflect fixation on a perinatal complication. From the point of view of prenatal psychology, it is clear that psychiatric concepts do not take enough account of the effects of a threatened prenatal existence on postnatal relationship to the world. This fact shows itself most clearly in psychiatric therapy. Also, in the case of schizophrenia, the synergy of pre-, peri- and postnatal stress factors is important for the later development of the illness. This was demonstrated in an empirical study by the German child psychiatrist Keppler (1979). In patients with schizophrenia, there was a combination of prenatal and birth trauma, emotional conflict in the family, and early disturbance of the child's contact with its environment.

The efforts now pursued for many years to find a genetic cause of schizophrenia have not led to any clear result. It has only been possible to distinguish the inheritance of a disposition toward "a certain developmental possibility of the personality." Thus, it seems sensible to me to include the observations of prenatal psychology in attempts to explain schizophrenic illnesses. As Fitzpatrick's perceptive study demonstrates, this approach is especially helpful when it comes to therapy. Recently, the Hungarian psychoanalyst and psychiatrist Jenö Raffai (1991, 1995, 1996) has developed a therapeutic model that assumes that schizophrenic patients are prenatally regressed. Here is a glimpse at Raffai's work:

> The young man standing opposite the wall reacts. He does not know that the room is his mother's body. The walls are his mother and at the same time the boundaries of his own body. He would like to break out of there but does not know how because he does not even know where he is. In the therapy, it is possible to get the birth-delivery process going and to understand it. At this point, he stops reacting and recognises that the room is the womb out of which he would like to step. . . . The 24-year-old patient stands on his head to act out his position before birth. Later he has the idea that he is under the influence of extra-terrestrial powers. He is a puppet who is dragged around, just a part of a huge machine. He is controlled by robots. During the therapy, I slowly become his surroundings. I am no longer a person but a machine, a robot. He is inside of me and I function organically with monotonous uniformity, like a machine. Everything happens with the same rhythm.
>
> Somehow something flows out of me into him that his body feels attracted to. Now he knows that he spreads his bodily sensations into me and that this represents the processes which occurred between his mother and his body. [1991, p. 268]

Fitzpatrick and Raffai are agreed that it is necessary in a supportive therapeutic context to achieve together with the patient a new, integrated birth, a birth that includes the psychological level. The Greek psychiatrist Maria Diallina (1987) has provided a very graphic description of this process as it occurred in the case of a Yugoslavian nurse who was very psychotic. The therapy involved working with clay. Here is an extract from the therapy report:

> The patient's desire to be reborn expressed itself in the image of a fish lying in air. It was alive and suffocating. It did not have any protective water around it. It had an enormous hunger which could be seen in its throat which seemed to be swallowing the whole world. This stood in stark contrast to the patient's "extreme flight from the world." To understand the dialect of this fish is the first sign of communication without space, without uterus, without water. The fish is lying on dry sand and is trying to breathe. The deep symbiosis of this process and the separation after the psychological birth became further apparent in the patient's transference: in her illness, the patient due to her passivity was only to be reached as an unborn fetus. The doctors had to visit her at home in order to get in touch with her. Shortly before her psychological birth she gave her therapist the last clay figure which she had made, a representation of the Turkish man murdered by neo-Nazis in Ulm. She explained that the Turk was now no longer an exile and blind. Death had freed him. He was no longer a foreign worker. (The figure, although dead, made a peaceful impression.) At this point, the patient had at last moved into sheltered accommodation and had for the first time in twenty years made contact again with her family in Yugoslavia. Later, after a successful "birth," the patient was able to demonstrate her new-found sense of boundaries even towards her psychotherapist and to leave her: "I do not need her any longer." [p. 228]

Very often, however, the psychotic patients' regression and efforts to be reborn do not lead to better contact with reality. Here is the example of a schizophrenic patient whose attempt to be reborn only ended in further searching for her lost umbilical cord, her "spender":

The patient stated that she had been dead and that since she had begun to live again, her "Spender" (German: *Spend*) was missing. How she had lost it, she could not say exactly. She assumed that she had died during an appendix operation and that afterwards "everything was different." Since then she was no longer just Martha Friedhof (= graveyard) but also an actress who had to search among her roles for who she really was. . . . What she was still missing in order to be her real self again was the "Spender." This is a sort of life force. . . . "Spender" is something like that which can be added again to the bodies of those who have not got it by blood transfusion. However, it has to be blood from others if it is to help. [Rausch 1988a, p. 14]

ANOREXIA NERVOSA

In my opinion, the perinatal roots of anorexia nervosa are little recognized. Typically, these patients develop a deep conflict about their feminine identity during puberty and it is not possible for them to find a starting point for their own independent existence by identifying with their mother. It will be easier to understand this difficulty if the findings of the American psychoanalyst Eva Jones (1985) are confirmed. In the majority of her patients, the mother had rejected the pregnancy and had tried in various ways to hide it. In numerous cases, the mother had tried to achieve this by going hungry. Jones gained the impression that the anorexia patients treat themselves in the same way that their mother had done in the first stages of the pregnancy. According to her report, an explanation of this connection had helped the majority of her patients to resolve their unhealthy symbiosis with negative aspects of their mother. In addition, Jones offered breathing techniques with which several patients were able to relive and sort out their experience of prenatal rejection as well as of their birth.

8

From Fetus to Adult:
Pre- and Perinatal Aspects of
Developmental Psychology

PROSPECTS

The examples in the previous chapters show us that our
earliest experiences remain alive and active within each of
us. Our whole existence is based on the vitality and the
dynamic experiences of our very beginning. This period is
physically and psychologically the foundation of our life and
our experience and of our relationship to the world. Every
new horizon in life is a transcendence and at one and the
same time a transformation and preservation of earlier
horizons. The vitality of the unborn child is to be seen again
in the vitality and elation of the suckling infant, then to be
assimilated and refreshed in the joyful existence of the

toddler and youngster. Each stage of life has its own specific forms of expression and possibilities of relationship and of pleasure. The psychotherapeutic situation allows us to observe how elements of earlier stages are preserved within us simply because conflict caused them to be repressed or split off. Then they take no further part in the processes of development and as a result continue to exist within us more or less unchanged. Freud spoke of the *Überlebseln*—"the bits that survive" (see Masson 1986, p. 279). We have got to know some of these "bits," for example, in childhood anxieties and in the formation of other symptoms.

Prenatal psychology offers us a new approach to understanding ourselves and our world. The fact that we have two different experiences of life, one in the prenatal and the other in the postnatal world, radically influences our understanding of ourselves and of our life. Humans have apparently always possessed a concept of a present world and of a world beyond. Every expression of human culture has been shaped by this assumption. In the course of history, the present and the beyond have been related to one another ever anew. We know that the relationship of the individual to the collective has its own history. Because the general existential crisis and social incoherence of the Middle Ages led to much fear, recourse to the primordial world beyond was all the stronger and governed people's attitudes to life. Only in this way was it possible to evade the real misery. The improved quality of life and the increased stability of our social structures reduce the pressure on us to search for support in a world beyond. The nineteenth century belief in progress and the certitude that a social utopia could be realized caused the projection of our original, prenatal world in religion to wane, so much so that Nietzsche, in speaking of the death of God, could proclaim the demise of this wish fulfillment as a cultural factor. The decline in the religious symbolization of human experience marked the birth of the discovery of the unconscious and the recognition that the otherworld was nothing other than the prenatal phase of our own existence.

Instead of the Fall and the expulsion from Paradise, we have Nietzsche's nihilism and Heidegger's *Geworfenheit* (*Translator's note:* literally, "having-been-whelped-ness"—a word derived by Heidegger from a word normally used to speak about the birth of animals). With this concept, Heidegger highlights our existential displacement and the animality of our having been born. Just as in Freud, where that intrinsic element of our earthly existence, fear, results from the primitive fact of our birth, so in Heidegger, it results from our *Geworfenheit*. Along with this development, our religious experience changed. The infantile belief in God the Father and the Mother of God, which had been shaped by the dilemma of the Middle Ages, became less potent and the way was opened to new forms of religious experience that are not based on the projection of infantile feelings. This cultural transition is closely linked to the discovery of prenatal psychology, which many artists, such as Dali and Klee, and writers, such as Beckett, were aware of. Conversely, one can also understand the discovery of the unborn child within us as an expression of the cultural transition.

If the perils and immeasurable human suffering of previous times were the main reasons for splitting off our pitiful existence here from a heavenly existence beyond, the discovery that the world beyond is nothing other than a projection of a part of our own biography offers us the chance to gain a holistic view of ourselves and the world. The unhealthy split between this world and the next has been and still is a fundamental concept of our culture and how it

in turn has defined countless aspects of our social life—
above and below, right and wrong, good and bad, master
and servant. Our individual and collective life were only
conceived of and experienced within this harmful derange-
ment between an idealized, heavenly world and a pitiful
postnatal existence. In previous times, the beginning of life
was for the majority of children a terrible ordeal. The
appalling statistics for perinatal and infant mortality are sad
evidence of this. The improvement in the conditions under
which children develop that has occurred in the last century
has been a prerequisite of our ability to suspend the
projection of our primitive, infantile feelings (DeMause
1979a). Thus, we have become more aware of the child, the
infant, and the unborn child within us.

This chapter is intended to encourage this deepening of
awareness. The long-term effects of our prenatal experience
on our postnatal existence will be illustrated and described
to help the unity and continuity within our life to become
apparent. It is unavoidable that these will only be provisional
considerations and comments intended to define some new
aspects of the psychology of culture that prenatal psychology
has uncovered. I am convinced that the manifestation of the
two basic phases of our life, the pre- and postnatal, within
our individual and collective psychological development can
always be changed and take on new forms. It represents the
starting point for the formation of both our individual and
our culturally determined emotional identity.

PRE- AND PERINATAL ASPECTS OF PSYCHOLOGICAL
DEVELOPMENT FROM INFANT TO ADOLESCENT

The helplessness we experience at the beginning of our life
makes us search for traces of our first, intrauterine security

within the family. On the one side, our picture of our parents is distorted by devotion, honor, and the idea that they are saints and wonderful. On the other side, our picture of our parents contains the dark aspects of fear, panic, and terror. In the early relationship to the infant, the parents try to restore the bliss of prenatal coziness by rocking, warmth, care, and devotion. The relationship thrives upon the archaic force of this desire. At the same time, depending on the particular culture and the brutality of the upbringing, feelings of helplessness and subjection to the parents' strength are impressed upon the child. Allowing the child to scream or to go hungry, disrespect of the child's needs, and beatings form the basis for the development of an authoritarian, aggressive adult who has learned that there is no security in this world, only derision and servitude.

Because humans are always born too early, our first extrauterine year is completely dominated by the desire to reproduce prenatal security. Growing out of this biological dependency during our second year of life corresponds to a psychological birth that has been described by the psychoanalyst Margaret Mahler (1978). The child gains control over his own mobility, can move himself around, begins to crawl and to walk, can eat by himself, separates himself from his mother's breast, and learns to control his toilet. In cases of conflict, the trauma of separation that occurred at birth can reappear in the child's tantrum attacks as it fights for its own individuality. During toilet training as the child learns to hold in, let go, and push out, he can relive and, under good conditions, also learn to cope with part of his birth experience. As the child becomes able to control his toilet behavior, he also becomes master of his own birth. He gets the confirmation that he brought himself into the world just as he can bring his toilet into the world. Psychoanalysis pointed early on to the connection in our experience between defecation and birth.

In his third year, the child gains social mobility. He or she appears as the little boy or little girl in the family and is, so to speak, born socially. This birth is then confirmed when the family recognizes that the child is mature enough to go to kindergarten. The child is in a peculiar phase of transition—he or she is already a social being but still feels protected and supported by the primary relationships within the family. The memory of the primal separation that occurred at birth appears here in the form of the danger related to the gender identity, which the child has just managed to achieve as little boy or little girl. Children recognize just how small and helpless they still are as they take their first steps into society. All this can be dealt with as the child learns about his or her own body. Vagina and penis can become the pledge and the proof of a new, social identity. However, in idealized reconditioning, they can also become ways of fleeing into prenatal security. The vagina becomes the proof of an archaic identity with the mother, a being at one with the secret of concealment, and the penis becomes a symbol of the umbilical cord and proof of prenatal omnipotence and union. When the birth trauma is reactivated, the vagina becomes the trigger for feelings of loss, injury, and the possibility of being captured and devoured. And because the penis is small, it leads to feelings of weakness and fear of being damaged. But when it is changed into the aggressor, it also becomes a means of piercing and destroying.

In the fourth and fifth year of life, the child completes his or her emancipation from the womb of the family and gains connection with social reality. This process is just the same sort of fundamental step toward maturity as puberty is and is connected somatically with physical transformations in the so-called first *Gestaltwandel,* a change in the shape and body proportions. This is actually the second *Gestaltwandel* because the first is the change from infant to child. The child is now strong enough for social autonomy and is capable of confronting his parents with feelings of love and hate—at least when they protect and accompany the child in a way appropriate to the conditions of his age and support his developmental needs. Then the child can successfully develop to school maturity when he has to a degree internalized his socially independent relationship to his parents as his own conscience and ideal and has thereby emancipated himself from direct parental care and leadership.

This internalization signifies the restoration of the double world on a new level. Through a psychological transformation, the early parental world becomes an inner world, and as a result an internalized arena for certain feelings and actions then comes into operation. This step has its original model in the experience of the two worlds after birth. The prenatal world becomes an internally represented inner world for the infant after birth. He seeks to find this again as his ideal self, as psychoanalysis expresses it, in his relationship to his mother. The developmental step from infant to small child is one of the first comparable changes in which the infant's world becomes an inner world that is sought again in conflict situations as a regressive reference point in the relationship to the parents. The small child still has the world of the infant in his memory as an internal reference point to which he can return in a situation of conflict. We know that a child can stop walking and speaking and start wetting and dirtying himself again in a conflict situation. That is, he becomes an infant again. In the distress and uncertainty of his present situation, the child conjures up the security of a previous stage of development. The same is true of the infant who, for example, refuses to be fed out of protest against some unpleasantness, and then retreats to the illusion of an imaginary prenatal sustenance through the umbilical cord.

When there is not enough support from the parents, it is possible that the child is unable to cope with the individuation steps in the fourth and fifth year of life. When the child's experience of the father is one of fear, then the temptation to regress to the comfortable existence provided by the mother can pull the child back to the coziness of the first, prenatal phase of life. The parents can let the transition to school with the accompanying experiences of helplessness and immaturity seem to be positively and negatively overwhelming. Fear of the next step in development actualizes early individuation fears, as far back as a possible birth trauma. However, there is also the possibility that during a new phase of self-discovery one can rely on earlier strengthening experiences of self-actualization, even the feelings of triumph and victory of the first big adventure of a successful birth. A new world is conquered by birth and the earlier one is internalized. Every phase of development is concerned with a new, constructive ordering of one's identity and relationship to the world, that is, a constructive transformation and primal experience of the two worlds, the prenatal world and the postnatal world.

Within the self (*Ich-Gefühl*), the earlier identity is overthrown but at the same time conserved to the extent that it is the foundation and starting point for the new stage of life and contains the possibilities of further development. Psychoanalysis describes this broader part of the personality, that is, the personality that one is and always was, as the self. In prenatal life, the *Ich* and the self are still coexistent, whereas after birth they can begin a creative interplay (Graber 1978a). The internal communication between the *Ich* and the self can get lost because of the traumatic upheavals in development. One also speaks popularly of losing one's self, of losing one's roots, and even of alienation. Fragments of the self can remain in projection because of traumatic stress or culturally determined limits set on development. Then they can be connected to political institutions and persons as the *Ich*-ideal. This prevents the true discovery of the self.

At latency or school age, a child is still dependent on the parents and the restricted social group of neighbors, acquaintances, and school. He uses his new possibilities and proficiency to gain experience of the cultural inheritance of the world in which he lives. In some cases the two worlds, that of school and that of the parental home, can harmonize. With a certain credulity, the communicated issues are taken in and transferred into the child's own growing expertise. Children in the so-called latency phase can appear less self-reliant and more dependent than at the beginning of their individuation to child. The French psychoanalyst Gérard Mendel (1972) describes, for example, the situation in his country where children enter a very strict school system at the age of 6 and are made dependent and, in his opinion, held in an incomplete individuation. Cultural influences are effective (here) in a direct and unbroken way. C. G. Jung also saw the child before puberty as living in a symbiosis with his or her parents and was of the opinion that the child achieved a psychological birth only at puberty. However, I have the impression that children today have more autonomy and freedom and make frequent use of the cultural and social possibilities for their development.

Puberty is then the time of powerful biological and

psychological development and personal maturation. The ability to leave one's childhood behind is predetermined by the mastering of earlier steps of individuation from unborn child to infant, then to toddler, and then to childhood. Our culture demands a very high level of autonomy and thus the developmental task posed by puberty has become more comprehensive and requires a recapitulation, at least at a symbolic level, of previous orientations to life. It is in this way that the foundations of a new life as an adult are determined, making decisions based on one's own personal experience. Because we all have clear memories of puberty, it is the example that best allows us to observe the dynamics of the processes of human individuation.

Through maturation, the adolescent loses his foothold in childhood. He falls out of his familiar world. The only experience of a place apart from this world is of the world before that of childhood, that is of the world of the infant, baby, and unborn child. The primal experience of the two worlds communicated by birth and arrival in the postnatal world influences the approach to the confusing experience of biological maturation and the lack of confidence with the various aspects of adult roles. As a result, adolescents always retreat to a place, symbolic of early security, in order to dismantle their old identity as child and to construct a new one appropriate to adult life. As various adolescent subcultures demonstrate, this place of transformation, full of prenatal symbolism, can take various forms. It can be the place used by a social group; it can also be the place defined by fantasy, by reading, by films, or by one's own poetry. Since adolescent individuation or becoming adult is a central theme of cultural creation, adolescents can find unlimited inspiration here. Our ways of going through puberty are multifarious and individual, as opposed to tribal culture where the social group sets a strict framework for the processes of maturation. The birth of the adult *Ich* results from a fresh and creative application of the primal experience of the two worlds. Only an internal appropriation of one's preceding life from the very beginning provides the basis and freedom required for the step to independent existence and relationships without the necessity of always seeking in others a protective, parental figure.

The adolescent individuation process is an essential stimulus for further cultural development. The "almost adult" is already acquainted with his culture's traditions and values. In the regression stimulated by his biological maturation, all these cultural experiences are checked once again against the desires and fantasies of early and earliest childhood. Spurred on by any incongruity with the earliest psychological foundations, the new adult can come to set completely new creative aims. There is the possibility of a process of transformation of the acquired personal identity in an advanced phase of life that is unknown to us in the animal kingdom.

The important American psychoanalyst Kurt R. Eissler (1978) goes so far as to maintain that, without what Freud called the two-stage development of sexuality, that is, the oedipal phase and puberty, mankind would not have developed beyond the invention of the hand flint. The significance of puberty is dependent on how convincing the ideas communicated during the latent phase are. If, due to cultural change or technological innovation, the ideals set by the parents have become unrealistic, then puberty becomes a very significant time of reorientation for the adolescent. Depending on how successful the new formulations are, the adult's inner and external worlds can correspond much

better to one another. The external world can then become
the place where the person's desires and needs that have
become clear during the experience of puberty can be
realized.

After life's aims and tasks have been achieved and
realized in the middle period of life, mid-life is then a
further phase of transition in self-understanding. Again
here, this step in individuation is based on a new integration
of the inner and outer worlds. This mid-life individuation
was the main concern of Jung's work. A return to one's
origins may be necessary for a person to align his previous
personal experience with life's new perspective.

So far, the turning points and steps of individuation were
the main topics under consideration. Now we must visualize
development to be a process of human self-constitution, a
progressive exchange and processing of previous experience. This becomes clear when certain elements are not
integrated because of traumatic interruptions in the continuous processes of development. Psychoanalysis demonstrated this in the example of the hindered development
from infant to child, in the example of incomplete resolution of the Oedipus complex. It is clear in the case of
someone who cannot come to terms with fear of the father,
sibling rivalry, or fear of the mother, so that his pattern of
life and behavior is determined by the people involved in his
conflict. This is also equally true for failure in early phases of
self-realization. I have already mentioned how peculiarities
in prenatal experience or birth can undercut much of our
development in later life.

When conflict is less apparent or more strongly repressed, then a child can accommodate the undercurrents
of his personality in the games and interactions that society
offers him. Thus, children's games can be understood as

opportunities for continuous integration of previous experience, even those from life before birth. However, more than this, prenatal life and birth are to a certain extent primal symbols, and a clear perception of our personal identity is dependent on their reenactment. Thus, children's games have a pre- and perinatal component. Catching or tag repeats the perinatal interplay between liberation and captivity. Hide-and-seek repeats the interplay between prenatal security and being expected in the world outside. Competition in general repeats the fundamental confirmation that one has been victorious in the elementary struggle of birth. All dramatic games and stories repeat in various ways the basic themes of the fairy tales about a journey to another world to find the treasure of regeneration, a return to life's beginning, or a battle with a dragon as a repetition of birth. Society offers innumerable patterns to live out again and again and to integrate one's own experience of individuation. Even in games governed by rules, it is always a question of renewed attempts to process the experience of birth, which is registered in our deepest unconscious. The fact that the themes and patterns involved in games are limited reflects the limits imposed by the human birth experience.

CHILDREN'S GAMES AND STORIES—FROM THE WILD THINGS TO SUPERMAN AND E.T.

A comprehensive analysis of children's games and stories to show how they present and repeat primal experiences is not possible here. Because it is so well known, the children's book *Where the Wild Things Are* by Maurice Sendak (1987) has been taken as an arbitrary example. It contains the typical formula for individuation that can be found in practically every children's story: damage or destruction—regression to another world to gain regeneration—and then return. The book about the wild things is about little Max's temper. His mother has rejected him because of it. His relationship to his mother becomes disturbed and he must go to bed without anything to eat. His regression is reflected in the transformation of his bedroom into a prenatal symbol, a forest. This theme is then underlined by a journey in a ship to another world. Meeting a dragon is a symbolic repetition of the danger of birth. In another world, he then meets the "wild things," that is, his own infantile or prenatal rage, to which he forms a healing, regenerative relationship. All the "primal ones" make an incredible noise together and display their fury. Thus strengthened, he can discharge the trauma he has experienced from his mother onto the wild things and sends them to bed without food. In his own world where he is in control, he can compensate for the humiliation suffered in his relationship to his mother. As a result of this, his return home—where the supper is still waiting for him—becomes possible.

An example of a game that very clearly symbolizes birth is "Petzi," based on the children's comic story. In the middle of the playing board, there is an island on which there is an octopus covered with picture cards depicting meadows and shrubs. At the edge of the board, there are pictures of houses with closed doors. Apart from numbers, the die also has a picture of an octopus. When this turns up, then a card is removed from the island and the octopus is gradually freed. The aim is by correct die numbers to land at the house pictures. Then the door has to be opened to escape from the octopus. Just like the small child in the "Petzi" stories, one has to escape from the evil octopus–birth mother and find refuge in the good house-mother.

Apart from games and stories, the annual fair is a further example of a controlled form of regression. With swings, carousels, roller coasters, and ghost trains, it provides numerous pre- and perinatal sensations, both pleasant and terrifying. The reader can fill in the details from his own experience.

Hero comics confront us very clearly with the derivatives of early experience. "Superman" is a good example. At the beginning of Superman's life, there is a traumatic birth catastrophe and he loses his parents; Superman comes from Krypton, a planet in deep space that was destroyed by a horrific catastrophe (Kupperberg 1980). Just as Otto Rank described it, the hero Superman represents the one who is free from fear and who tries to overcome an especially difficult birth. The birth is repeated and remedied in his various, superhuman tasks. Crime and emergency actualize the primal catastrophe of birth and are mastered once more by Superman's recourse to fetal omnipotence, especially shown in his ability to fly, an important prenatal symbol. When there is an alarming report of a catastrophic crime, then the regressive transformation of the journalist Clark Kent into Superman takes place—always in a telephone booth, symbolic of connection to another world. Thus, Superman remains the eternal adolescent.

A more complicated example of the handling of perinatal experience triggered by an actual conflict is provided by one of the most successful films of all time, *E.T.* The father of the 6-year-old boy has left his family because of marital problems. Understood from the point of view of prenatal psychology, a longing for the security of the prenatal world surfaces in the child. This is expressed by the fact that he suddenly gains contact with an extraterrestrial being, E.T., who becomes his companion. E.T. can be understood as symbolizing the placental, prenatal companion. The restitution is ended by a revived experience of birth in which the disappearance of the prenatal companion is repeated— E.T. is picked up by a spaceship. Afterward, the small boy can face the parental conflict. The possibility of a new father appears in the last scene of the film. The decisive psychological point is that the loss of the father repeats the as yet unresolved loss of security experienced at birth. Because the boy regresses to the security of the prenatal relationship and is thus strengthened, he becomes able to withstand the terrors of birth. He becomes able to cope with the individuation toward more autonomy which has been made necessary by the parental conflict.

It is hoped that these various examples have made it clear that our unconscious is always actual and present or, expressed in another way, that the whole of our life's experience is always with us and that we must bring this into new balance in ever new movements of individuation. The original experience of the two worlds is a constitutive element of this. As a result, our concern is always with finding a new balance between these two worldviews. Taking the example of E.T., that means that the father was something like heaven for the boy, the representative of the other, prenatal world. When this heaven collapsed as he lost his father, he first had to check again internally the primal experience of his original world in order to be able to stand the duality of the inner and external realities.

9

Dying and Becoming: The Cultural Manifestations of Pre- and Perinatal Experience

OVERVIEW OF PRE- AND PERINATAL SYMBOLISM IN THE PROCESS OF CULTURAL DEVELOPMENT

Mankind has always been marked by a nostalgia for its origins, a nostalgia that makes new beginnings possible and that is expressed in myth and ritual. One of the oldest epics ever written, the epic of Gilgamesh, deals with a journey to the underworld to get the Herb of Life, which guarantees freedom from death. This fabulous-mythical region, which produces such precious, healing goods, is represented in the prenatal symbols of the primal cave, the primal ocean, and the tree of life. To a certain extent, these are symbolic representations of the primal experience of the security of the uterine cave, of swimming in the amniotic fluid, and of the well-being and health produced by placental nourishment. By experiencing the security of the uterus, the protection of the fluids, and the nurturing and nourishing tree, a person can get back in touch with his prenatal, primal experience and can then form new images of it within his culture. The journey to another world, to the tree of life, and submergence in the primal ocean are images that communicate the actualization of prenatal experience.

A continuous thread through human development appears to be the expansion of consciousness, the process of maturing away from instinctive forms of experiencing and behaving. This development of consciousness leads to a confrontation with mortality that itself reflects questions about life's beginning.

The very first human cultures attempted to deal with the fear of death with the idea of rebirth. Ever since the Stone Age, many burial rituals use the fetal position. According to this soothing concept, death is simply a return to the fetal state, a return that is then followed by rebirth. All rituals at the turning points of life, in particular puberty, also follow the pattern of this basic model.

The child dies, enters a sort of fetal state of waiting, and is then born again as an adult. All rites of passage follow this pattern, even those of the heroes of myth and fairy tale. In every critical situation, one enters another world in which precious goods are to be obtained. Then a renewing, symbolic, social rebirth follows.

Seen psychologically, the return to prenatal origins makes it possible for a person to separate himself from previous instinctive behavior and relationships, and this is experienced as a death. It then allows creativity and the production of new combinations and connections. Perhaps one can imagine the prenatal mode of functioning of the psyche as free-floating between feelings of desire and ideas of fulfillment, something like what we already know from people in psychosis, from children's experience, and from our own dreams. According to my interpretation, regression to prenatal, primal experience followed by return to the normal world, but experienced then in a new way, represents a fundamental condition for human self-discovery, a "narcissistic transformation." What is meant here is initiation, which is the selection and ordination, controlled by particular customs, of a novice into a state of life or age group (in particular, the introduction of youth in primitive tribes into the circle of men or women), a process of transformation determined by the pattern of "dying and becoming" that allows the reproduction of a whole on a new level. From the primal experience of the two worlds, the prenatal and the postnatal, a person can always approach the outside world from a new and secure distance and at the same time make the outside world into the place where his imaginary desires can be realized. Because of our premature birth, the two worlds stand in a dramatic tension to one another, and I understand the creative use of this basic experience of the two worlds to constitute an essential element of cultural development. The helplessness that we experience at the beginning of postnatal life continuously feeds the desire to construct the world according to prenatal conditions as a realm of security, protection, and unending, magically communicated nourishment. These characteristics alone make it clear that essential elements of our cultural creations and efforts are intended to communicate this primary security again to us.

Religion provides explanations about why the paradise

we originally experienced was lost and communicates to us in cult-symbolic ways something of the primary proximity of our earliest beginnings and of nurture in a divine, primal being. From the very outset, religion comforts us about the limited nature of our existence with the promise of a return to the beginning. Political structures are also full of prenatal symbolism. The social role of the leader may have its biological prototype in instinctive behavior of the pack toward its leader. However, when the leader is dressed up by a culture as a king, then the insignia of prenatal-fetal omnipotence proclaimed in the coronation ceremony become decisive (Gehrts 1966b). But even our technological innovations and utopias are influenced by the fascination of trying to realize in this world some of the qualities of our prenatal existence. The effortless movement in our modern transportation systems can be associated to being carried and held in the prenatal situation, and modern information and news communications systems provide something of the prenatal enjoyment of limitless communication and an experience of proximity that transcends all boundaries.

Also, it appears that in sports in the last hundred years completely new areas of narcissistic "reanimation" providing dramatic possibilities of deep, regressive experiences have developed. Whether it be flying, diving, jumping, or other bodily experience, the reconnection with prenatal, primal pleasure might be essential in some hidden way. If, as I assume, the dangerous and life-threatening moments of primal experience are sometimes translated unconsciously into wars and structures of totalitarian domination, a deeper understanding of these connections within our experience becomes even more significant.

Only research on these phenomena on a much broader basis can determine the possibilities and limits of prenatal psychological concepts. No matter how strange some of the perspectives and conclusions hinted at here may seem, experience in psychotherapy does lead to the conclusion that pre- and perinatal and postnatal, preverbal experiences do continue to live on within us all. That is true for us as individuals and as members of social groups. We always experience the world in the light of all of our life's experiences, even our prenatal ones. Yes, even these can provide the roots of our deepest desires and pleasures, just as the experience and mastering of birth is the starting point of our ability to achieve ever fresh, elementary progress. In the following section, the cultural processing of pre- and perinatal experience is described using several examples. The presentation is rather a sketch intended to stimulate further considerations and the search for personal examples.

A PRIMARY THEME OF HUMAN CULTURE—
THE JOURNEY OF THE SHAMAN

Ethnological research in the last hundred years has informed us very well about the nature and function of the shaman's journey among primitive peoples. A shaman is for many primitive peoples the medicine man and the oracle who maintains contact with invisible spirits. Often he is also the leader during the initiation of young men. He reveals to them the secrets of nature and the rules by which a man must live. When a person becomes ill or a group has a crisis, the shaman goes on an inner journey to reclaim the lost health or welfare of the group. This always includes a transfer into another world beyond, whereby the change from the one world into the other is often induced by a crash, a fall, or by being swallowed, and in visual experience usually leads through a door and then an underground passage or tunnel that is secured by guards or wild animals. Frequently the journey to the other world is connected with altered states of consciousness and identity. Typically there are experiences of dying, of dismembering, and of reanimation and rejuvenation. Archetypical, healing experiences occur in the other world. This is followed by return to this world and the demonstration of special powers obtained through the journey, whether it be the ability to heal or to perform some other task.

Uterine symbolism is very evident in the reports that shamans have given of their experiences. The following example from a modern shaman journey shows this:

> I moved forwards in a dark and narrow place and found . . . a completely new cave. Concentric circles of light and darkness opened up around me and seemed to carry me. Actually I did not feel as though I was moving myself through the tunnel but rather as if it was moving past me. At first the rings were perfectly round but then changed their form . . . and opened up onto a view over a grey and weakly illuminated landscape . . . a lake across which I slid for a long time. I was able to observe exactly how the waves rose, foamed and moved underneath me. The tunnel which had brought me to this place sloped slightly, about 15 degrees. Now, however, the darkened sky over this lake drew me underground into another tunnel which led directly 90 degrees downwards and again it transported me through itself. Its walls consisted of the concentric circles of light and darkness I had already encountered. They were almost pulsating through me. It did not feel like falling but was rather a completely deliberate movement. [Harner 1982, p. 61]

If one accepts, as suggested, that the shaman's journey is a graphic reactivation and symbolization of pre- and perinatal experience, then the external form that the shaman's trance takes also becomes understandable. The drum he uses symbolizes the mother's heartbeat, and the rattle the noises from the digestive system, and both of these together induce the shaman's trance by mobilizing primal experience. Similarly, as Terence Dowling (1987, personal communication) has pointed out, the drum in the shamanistic ritual represents the placenta and the drumsticks the umbilical cord. Thus the use of the drum and rattle stimulates the trance, the fetal regression, which is then translated into images and pictures by the shaman during his journey. Here is a further example from the Eskimo culture:

> For the really great shamans, a path opens up directly from the house in which they call upon their helper-spirits. A road downwards through the earth when they are in a tent on the coast or downwards through the sea in the case of an igloo upon sea-ice. It is upon this road that the shaman is taken down without meeting the slightest obstacle. He slides, so to say, as if he is falling through a tube which fits so exactly around his body that he can control his progress by pushing against the walls and so does not really need to fall. This tube is held open for him by all the souls of his patrons until his journey brings him back to earth. [Harner 1982, p. 182]

The stories that people create for themselves in their fantasies also have roots in the tales told by the shamans about their journeys to other worlds. The theme of the shaman's journey to another world is to be found in fairy tales and myths as well as in many rituals. A journey back to our origins is a fundamental, collective-psychological theme because we all share the experience of the other, prenatal world. By moving into another world, by a journey to the heavenly and hellish origins of one's own existence, whereby a lost personal unity is reattained, or, expressed in psychological terms, by regression to the womb, prenatal, psychological sensibility is reconnected with the postnatal form of life, the prenatal self integrated with the postnatal, reality-oriented ego. This internal reconnection, which occurs in deep regression, goes hand in hand with a symbolic transition over the threshold of birth and the corresponding fantasies of horror, fright, and misery. Goethe gave this a classic formulation in *Faust*:

Yes, let me dare those gates to fling asunder,
Which every man would fain go slinking by!
'Tis time, through deeds this word of truth to thunder:
That with the height of Gods Man's dignity may vie!
Nor from that gloomy gulf to shrink affrighted,
Where Fancy doth herself to self-born pangs compel.
To struggle toward that pass benighted,
Around whose narrow mouth flame all the fires of Hell,
To take this step with cheerful resolution
Though Nothingness should be the certain, swift conclusion!
                                        [Goethe 1967b, p. 29]

Only when this fear is conquered is there a possibility of experiencing rejuvenation and new beginning. All heroes, whether in myth, fairy tale, or poem, have survived such journeys to another world. The central theme is always the symbolization of the female genitals in a door and cave or in an engulfing animal.

PUBERTY RITUALS AS A RETURN TO THE WOMB AND RENEWAL

In the initiation rituals that take place at the beginning of puberty, regression to the womb and rebirth as an expression of changing from one stage of life to another is often portrayed in a very realistic fashion. For example, in one ritual, the youths are born through a birth canal between two legs and then just like newborns cannot walk or speak. The ritual always begins for those who are going to be initiated with the abolition of their childhood world so that in regression the terrors of birth have to be experienced once more. The youths are then able to return after having been regenerated in a place symbolizing the prenatal world. Here is an example cited by the ethnologist Mircea Eliade (1988):

> Four days before the ceremony begins, the novices (those to be initiated among the Pangwe in Africa) receive a label which states: "Ordained to die." During the feast days themselves, they are given a drink which provokes nausea and the whole village shouts "You must die!" to whoever vomits. Then the novices are led into a house which is full of ants' nests. They are forced to remain in the house for some time and are exposed to terrible stinging during which the villagers shout "You will be killed. Now you must die!" The instructors lead the novices "towards death" to a hut in the jungle where they live for a whole month completely naked and in absolute isolation. They make their whereabouts known by use of a xylophone so that no one approaches them. At the end of the month, they are painted white and they are allowed to return to the village to take part in the dancing but they must sleep in the hut in the bush. . . . Only after a further three months, are they allowed to leave the bush. Among the

southern Pangwe, the ceremony is even more dramatic. A
ditch, which is intended to represent a grave, is covered with
a pottery figure, normally in the form of a mask. The ditch
also represents the belly of the cult deity and the novice must
step over it in order thus to signify their rebirth. [p. 62]

Depending upon the cultural context, the puberty
rituals can emphasize either the aspect of death, as in the
example above, or that of renewal and rebirth. Regression to
the womb can be portrayed more or less graphically. On this
subject, Eliade refers to the ethnologist Berndt. According
to the natives, the dance area in the Kunapipi ritual, which
is triangular, symbolizes the mother's womb:

When the neophytes exchange their camp for the ceremonial
area, it is imagined that they become holier and holier and
enter the primal mother. They reach her womb, a circular
place, just as it was at the beginning of time. When the ritual
has been completed, the mother lets them out. They leave
the round area and return once more to everyday life.
[p. 87] . . . One is surprised by the vehemence with which
the return to the womb is repeated. . . . The whole ceremony gives the impression that it has less to do with a ritual
death followed by resurrection as a total regeneration of the
initiand who goes back to the womb of the great mother and
is reborn from her. [p. 89]

On one decisive point, prenatal psychology goes further
than the descriptions offered by Eliade and the other
ethnologists: the rites of initiation are intended to show that
the developmental step of puberty and the first, major
transition in life that it reactivates, the transition from
prenatal to postnatal existence, are similar experiences. In
this way, it is intended that the youths are supported during

their adolescent phase of self-discovery. At the same time, the event is used to hold the group together and to communicate its fundamental view of reality. The marked effects and power of the initiation rituals are thus not—as the ethnologists believe—the result of abstract symbolization but rather of the reactivation of primal experience and its transformation into concrete, puberty rituals.

Whether from Africa or Asia, the descriptions of the rituals make it clear that the principal elements are uniform, because universal, primal experience manifests itself within the different cultural context and initiations. It seems essential that the dynamic of these various expressions of initiatory experience does not have just some archetypical root but is a reenactment and a creative use of individual, primal experience. To counter the impression that the conclusions here are based only on the opinions of Eliade, I now present the characteristics of puberty rituals as summarized by Vladimir Propp (1987), a Russian researcher of fairy tales:

> In one of the forms of the ritual, the initiand creeps through a construction which has the form of a terrifying animal. This terrible animal is represented by a special hut or a house constructed where there are already other buildings. The initiand is digested and then expelled as a new person. [p. 284]

The follow quotation illuminates the uterine symbol of the snake or dragon:

> We should not forget that in the ritual the emergence from the body of the snake is imagined as a second birth, the true birth of the hero. We have already seen how this was represented later in fairy tales by carrying him in a box and

placing it in water. This idea which is related to birth from a dragon goes back to the same sphere as the whole complex of battling with a dragon. The developmental stages can be schematised as follows: The one who has been born from the dragon (ie. the one who has gone through it) is the hero. In a further stage, the hero slays the dragon. The historical connection of these two themes leads to the following: the one born from the dragon is also the one who slays it. [p. 348]

A further piece of evidence for the perinatal aspects of puberty experiences is provided by the description of an old Greek puberty-initiation ritual from the social scientist Walter Burkert (1990):

Girls eligible for marriage are at first separated from the community and then a "meeting with Eros" is repeated in which she goes on a journey underground. There she encounters a snake, "the most terrible animal of all," which comes out of the darkness of the earth and which has always belonged to the cult of the dead. The death of the virgin is the birth of the woman. This is once again also represented in perinatal symbols. In the original version of the myth, when the virgins see the snake in a basket, they jump down the north face of the Acropolis to their death. [p. 48]

THE FAIRY TALE HERO'S JOURNEY TO THE BEYOND—SYMBOL OF LIFE'S BEGINNING: FROM TOM THUMB TO RAPUNZEL

Researchers are more or less agreed that fairy tales have basically two equally important roots. The first is to be found in the tales told by shamans about their journeys to the beyond and the second in the experience of puberty rituals.

Fairy tales are to a certain extent initiation expressed on the level of fantasy. Propp (1987) writes: "If one pictures everything that happens in an initiation and then relates it sequentially, one produces the sort of composition that magical fairy tales are based upon" (p. 452). As I have tried to make clear, however, the patterns of the puberty ritual and the shaman's journey are themselves drawn from the dynamic of reactivated pre- and perinatal experience. Central to both is the motif of regression to the womb and rebirth. In the shaman's journey this is imagined, and in the puberty ritual it is dramatized.

Sigmund Freud imagined that psychoanalysis would be able to transform religion and metaphysics into metapsychology. This is especially true in the case of fantasies contained in fairy tales. Early in the development of psychoanalysis, Otto Rank and Hans Sachs (1965) were able to demonstrate this persuasively. The development of the psychoanalytic study of fairy tales was hindered by conflict between the various schools of psychoanalysis. Whereas Freud traced the cultural projection and processing of early relationship to the father, Jung studied the projection of relationship to the mother in myths. Because the symbolism of regression to the womb and rebirth is central to fairy tales and because this is imperfectly reflected in the strict Freudian tradition with its overemphasis on the theme of the father, research into fairy tales dwindled. On the other hand, a strikingly large number of fairy tale interpretations appeared in Jungian analytical psychology, which does consider the symbolic and projective forms of regression to the womb and rebirth. In comparison, in strict Freudian psychoanalysis, there are only a few studies of the significance of fairy tales. Bettelheim's book, *The Uses of Enchantment* (1977), gives the impression that there is a profusion of psychoanalytic interpretations of fairy tales. In fact, Bettelheim, who himself criticizes Freud for having neglected the importance of the child's early relationship to the mother, simply fell back on Jungian interpretations indiscriminately and without stating his sources. As a result, his interpretations, despite all his reputed experience as a child analyst, have a patchwork character. It is about time that the tension between contradiction and correlation within the Freudian and Jungian interpretations of fairy tales was discussed. Because the pre- and perinatal roots of a child's first fears of his or her mother and father, as pointed out by Rank and Graber, have remained unrecognized by both traditions, prenatal psychology could be of great help here. It has demonstrated to what extent fairy tales in particular are determined by the projection of pre- and perinatal experiences.

Intensive study of fairy tales within the last two hundred years has made it possible to work out the principal characters within a fairy story. Walter Scherf (1982) has formulated psychological descriptions:

> Fairy tales are essentially stories with two parts. In the first part, the main figures as adolescents separate themselves from their parents in order to go their own way. The first partnership which they experience on their way to discovering themselves falls apart again because of their immaturity. An extraordinary effort is required—the theme of the second part—in order to prove one's self a reliable partner and to make a lifelong, enduring relationship. [p. xi]

In many fairy tales, an explicit connection is made between the experience of birth and the process of separation involved in puberty. In "Sleeping Beauty," the threat of death from the negative side of the mother during the birth is symbolized in the wicked fairy. The reactivation of this in puberty leads to a psychological, deathlike, prenatal regression represented in the state of sleep. The heroine's own desires for life, symbolized by the intrusion of the Prince, develop out of this regression. These desires overpower the obstructive wall of thorns, her vaginismus, which is a further symbolic repetition of her perinatal death wish.

In his book, *The Morphology of the Folktale*, Vladimir Propp (1975) proposed a basic formula that can be connected to ideas about psychological regression to the beginning of life in a quite cogent way. Here is a summary of his formula: The hero is injured, has a crisis, or is separated from his parents. He then gets involved in a discussion with an old man or an old woman (in whom one can see the figures of the early parents). After that, he liberates the image of the princess from the other (prenatal) world and thus proves himself to be a man. He then succeeds in some difficult tasks; for example he survives traveling great distances. According to Propp, this successful accomplishment of the tasks signifies that he can travel back and forth between the different worlds. I would put it this way: after the process of maturation, he is no longer threatened by his unconscious, the infantile, and the embryonal in his identity. Rather, on the contrary, his primal experience can now be integrated in a creative way with his experience of postnatal life into a single view of the world. In Rank's view, this would mean that he had overcome his birth trauma. When one sees it in this way, one can then understand that fairy tales are guided fantasy or shaman journeys that convey the fundamental experience of the reenactment of life's beginning during the transition from youth to adulthood. The experienced deficit is in the fairy tale and in reality the precondition for achieving a new stand in life. The dearth of sufficient space, oxygen, and nourishment experienced by the fetus at the end of the pregnancy is the precondition for the birth process, just as later the deprivation determined by the processes of maturation during adolescence and the loss of parental protection elicit and hasten the transition of puberty.

An example of the way in which the processes of maturation are expressed in the case of a premature birth is offered in the fairy tale "Tom Thumb." "Now it happened that the woman became ill and after seven months bore a child which was perfectly formed in all its parts but no bigger than a thumb" (Grimm and Grimm 1969, p. 148). Because of Tom's incompleteness, his process of maturation is marked by permanent reversion to the womb and rebirth: the hero disappears in an ear, in the folds of his father's suit, in a mouse's hole, and so on. Ultimately, he is swallowed by a cow that in turn is eaten by a wolf. In the well-known style of heroes, he finally frees himself again, albeit with the help of his father, who cuts the wolf open. I understand this supportive function of the father as symbolizing a positive relationship to the father, which is helpful when one goes through the dangers of deep regression. In the case of Tom Thumb, however, the yearning to get back to the beginning is so strong that he does not achieve a real independence. The fairy tale ends with the father's question: "Where on earth have you been?" to which Tom replies: "Ah, father, I was in a mouse's hole, in the belly of a cow and in a wolf's stomach. Now I will stay with you."

An equally incomplete maturation is portrayed in the fairy tale "The Three Snake Leaves." In this tale, a father can no longer nourish his only son. Thereupon, the son goes off into the world and marries a king's daughter. A condition of the marriage, however, is that if he is still alive when his wife dies, he must allow himself to be buried with her. And indeed, that is what happens. In the grave, he heals his wife with curative leaves that he has obtained from a snake. However, his wife proves to be evil and tries to drown him and to deceive him. A faithful servant saves him, once again with the help of the snake leaves. The king receives him again with honors and the evil princess is punished—she is put out to sea in a boat full of holes.

The fundamental deficiency is symbolized by the father's inability to nourish his only son. The prenatal regression, the task involved in the process of maturation, is contained in the condition set for the marriage—to allow himself to be buried alive with his dead wife. The womb symbolism in this story was identified very early by Freud. The snake and the healing leaves—symbols of the positive umbilical cord and placenta—appear in the critical situation of starvation in the grave. Through a further uterine regression, the recovery is again annulled by the second actualization of the image of the evil mother in the form of the unkindness of the woman. This time, it is an aspect of the positive image of the father in the form of the "faithful servant" that saves the son in a small boat. This takes place by means of the symbol of "umbilical reconnection"—the application of the snake leaves (symbol of the placenta). Nevertheless, because of the deficient negativity of the feminine elements, the maturation remains incomplete—a lasting marriage does not come about.

An example of a fairy tale that describes a prenatal injury indirectly is "Hans My Hedgehog." Because his father had wished it during the pregnancy, Hans is born in a hedgehog skin, symbol of his having been rejected. Again in this fairy tale, conflict in the parental home during puberty is the occasion for the reliving of the early rejection and a return to life in the forest, symbolic of uterine existence. There the hero gets a grip on himself again so that he is man enough to face the challenge and can win his bride.

The fairy tale of the "Devil with the Three Golden Hairs" shows how a good birth, symbolized by being born with the amnion over the head, can be the foundation for the ability to make single-minded transitions in life. The hero is a match for all the predicaments posed for him by his persecutory father.

"Rapunzel" is also concerned with prenatal injury. The mother is overcome by self-destructive yearnings for her own mother and before the birth is so consumed by her search for lamb's lettuce (Rapunzel) that she nearly dies. As a result, even in the womb Rapunzel comes under the spell of the image of an evil mother, which then dominates her later life. The mother's complete opposition to birth is reenacted in Rapunzel's incarceration in the tower—an image of return to the womb. The positive maternal elements are represented by the window and the positive intrauterine experiences by the golden hair. The love for the Prince signifies the power of sexuality and Eros in overcoming the birth trauma. Then the negative fixation on the birth trauma becomes operative once more in the transposition into the desert and the forest. However, this is then surmounted by the fact that Rapunzel herself has twins, a boy and a girl, symbolizing wholeness.

Also in the story of "Snow White," it is the latent prenatal death wishes of the mother and her death during the birth that traumatically determine Snow White's development and pose a deadly threat to her entrance into life as an adult woman. That the mother wishes a child "as white as snow, as red as blood, and as black as ebony" can be seen according to Odermatt (1987) as an anticipation of the "step-mother's attempts to kill Snow White. With the poisoned comb in her hair, the poisoned, red apple and the general intention that she should become white, that is, dead" (p. 30). The mother's ambivalent desire for a child impairs Snow White's fetal existence and is continued after her birth in the negativity symbolized by the stepmother. Again here it is the entrance into puberty, the blossoming of the young woman, that reactivates the primal trauma and induces the return to various places symbolizing uterine existence—the forest, the dwarves' cottage, and the glass coffin. Also in this fairy tale, in the end it is the power of sexual instinct, symbolized in the love of the Prince, that makes available the energy for further development.

In the fairy tale "Marienkind," it is obvious how contact with the first sexual emotions in puberty, represented by the pushing of a key into a lock, activates incestuous and dangerous prenatal feelings. The stimulus for the adventure of development at puberty is doubled—the Mother of God takes the child because the parents can no longer look after her but then she leaves the child alone again and goes on a journey. The girl opens the forbidden door, a fact made obvious later by the gold on her finger. As a punishment, she is placed in sleep and has to eke out a meager living in a hollow tree under the earth until a prince frees and marries her. The return to the prenatal mother is represented pictorially by the deep sleep, by being placed under the earth and in the wilderness, as well as by the fact that she has to creep into an old, hollow tree. This symbolization of the umbilical reconnection, the return to the tree of life elicits a revitalization and the discovery of a new identity as woman. In the fairy tale, this identity still has to contend with persecution by the "evil mother" but in doing so the Marienkind demonstrates the maturity she has gained.

ASPECTS OF BIRTH IN TALES ABOUT HEROES

Otto Rank (1909) extracts the "typical saga" from a synopsis of tales about heroes. With this, one can illustrate how the sagas attribute a completely different significance to the conditions pertaining at life's beginning than the one that we are used to. The rational approach to life, which has dominated the last two hundred years in our culture, minimized the significance of the early stages of life in order to strengthen belief in reason. Now, from the standpoint of deeper knowledge, prenatal psychology can evaluate the significance of life's earliest events anew. The typical saga leads us to the following picture:

> The hero is the child of most distinguished parents. Most often he is a prince. Various difficulties precede his concep-tion—for example, chastity or continual infertility or secret sexual intercourse between the parents because of a external prohibition or obstacle. During the pregnancy or even ear-lier, it is predicted in a dream or oracle that the child's birth poses some sort of a threat. Most often, it is the father who is in danger. As a result of this, on the instigation of the father or a person who represents him, it is decided that the new-born child should be killed or exposed. As a rule, the child is placed in a casket and put to water. Then he is rescued by animals or simple folk (shepherds) and suckled by an female animal or a simple woman. As a adult, the child after a very eventful journey finds his distinguished parents again, takes revenge upon his father, is then recognised and achieves greatness and fame. [p. 61]

From the point of view of prenatal psychology, the following interpretation is possible. In this context only the prenatal elements will be emphasized. The idealization of the parents and their elevation into another world are symbol and idealization of the prenatal world of relationship to the parents with their splendor and magical omnipotence. The power and significance of hierarchical, social institutions come from the projection of this prenatal relationship with the parents: kings and queens bask in the splendor of a prenatal superworld and as a result suggest fetal security. However, in the saga, this is threatened by parental conflict and difficulties in which I see the symbolization of prenatal trauma. The prenatal, parental conflict results in a birth that breaks the continuity of the hero's life. The birth then leads to exposure, to loss of roots and relationships. This negative experience degrades the parents and the psychological misery affects the hero's developmental chances. The Hero is one who, despite this impairment, gains social status. This happens most often when he returns the humiliation that he suffered at the beginning of his life, assuming the reverse role in deeds of revenge and murder usually committed against the father.

The patriarchal background of this typical saga is obvious in the fact that conflict with the mother is transferred to the father and the son "makes himself" through his own prowess. Above all, the ability to fight is endorsed and it is from this that the person obtains the strength of his identity. This is particularly clear in the case of Heracles, whose overcompensating, masculine style of life finds its roots in the disastrous hostility of the goddess-mother Hera toward his birth: "Then she hurried to Thebes and squatted with crossed legs in front of Alkmenes' door, her clothes fastened in knots and her fingers clenched together, so that the birth of Heracles was delayed" (Ranke-Graves 1985, p. 411).

This birth trauma was then amplified by the trauma of exposure after birth and a breast-feeding trauma: "Hera picked Heracles up and bared her breast on which Heracles began to suck with such force that in her pain she threw him away from her. A trace of milk shot into the heavens and became the Milky Way. 'This little monster!' shouted Hera but Heracles was already immortal" (p. 415).

Hera is then supposed to have forcefully thrown the little Heracles onto the floor. This maternal aggression is repeated once more at the end of his first year of life. Hera sent three snakes but Heracles strangled them and thereby overcame the negative, maternal power. These events make Heracles' exaggerated masculinity and his body-oriented attitude understandable. The lion skin that protected him can be understood as the protective coating of the uterus, as a symbol of positive prenatal experience that the hero has as a reference to his power. With regard to this motif and that of invulnerability, which is connected to it, Rank spoke of a "permanent uterus."

It becomes clear from the saga of Heracles with what complexity the events surrounding a hero's birth are connected with the things that determine his destiny as an adult in a particular cultural setting and limit the possibilities of individual, personal development. The heroic life of Heracles is marked by battles against monsters and dragons, signifying heroic liberation from tendencies toward dependence upon the mother. As in other Greek hero sagas, the transition from a matriarchal to a patriarchal conception of culture is reflected here. For this reason, the Jungian analyst Neumann, (1956) spoke of a "Dragon-fight mythology" (p. 86).

THE ROOTS OF MYTH

From the point of view of prenatal psychology, a certain creative expression of the basic experience of two worlds is reflected in myths. From our present point of view, the myth maker still lived in projection. That is, his emotions appeared to him as imaginative pictures and because of this his conception of life and the world remained that of a child. This can be seen quite clearly in the behavior of the Homeric heroes; in times of conflict, they were not overcome by conflicting feelings but rather fell into a regressive trance. They did not feel but rather hallucinated or imagined something we also know well from childhood experience. An example is the quarrel between Agamemnon and Achilles over a trophy that Achilles is refused. Offended, he responds by retreating. He sits down by the sea in tears and pleadingly stretches his arms out to his mother:

"Mother, since you bore me to live only for a short time,
The Olympians should definitely guarantee me honour,
Zeus, the Mighty Thunderer! Now, however, he honours me
    not in the slightest!
Truly! The son of Atreus, the despotic Agamemnon, has
    disgraced me. He has taken and has in his possession my
    trophy which he personally took away from me!"
He spoke thus, shedding tears. And his august mother, who
    sat in the depths of the salty flood with his aged father,
    heard him.
And quickly she emerged out of the grey sea like a mist
And sat down in front of him, the shedder of tears,
Stroked him with her hand, spoke a word and named(?) it
    forth:
"Child, why do you cry?"
                          [Homer 1979, p. 14]

This is followed by an attempt to bring order into his confused emotions. It is important to notice how mythical experiences moves back and forth between the actual situation and trancelike imagination. This makes it understandable that we can conceive of mythical events as a sort of projected psychology or, to use the early psychoanalytical formulation, as a collective dream. Primal experiences express themselves in a symbolic form in myths in the same way as in individual dreams.

One of the most widespread mythological themes is that of the Tree of Life, in Germanic mythology, the World Ash, Yggdrasil. This Tree of Life guarantees the existence of the world. It connects the middle of the earth with heaven and gives the "Food of Life." In critical situations, the image of the tree can become a sanctuary. Terence Dowling (1990) has demonstrated that the various mythological stories concerning the Tree of Life quite accurately reflect the unborn child's experience of its placenta. Some of the ritual tree symbols have very explicit placental characteristics. Also the Tree of Life, described in alchemy, has this character: it is to be found in the primal ocean, it is full of blood, and when it falls the end of the world is at hand. In many illustrations, the trunk of the tree of life has a spiral structure, which can be seen to be the reflection of the serpentine umbilical cord.

Another symbol of prenatal experience is that of the magic rope that connects heaven and earth together. This motif is present in many cultures but is especially well expressed in India. The cosmic threads hold the universe together. At the end of the world, the threads will be cut and the universe will dissolve. Something similar is found in Homer's picture of the "golden chain" by means of which Zeus was able to pull all things to himself. As the following report from Mircea Eliade (1960) shows, the regressive trance is also able to reactuate primal experience: "During the initiation of the medicine man and brought about by the ritual singing, a rope appears in his body which allows him to draw fire out of his body, to climb up trees and to travel into heaven" (p. 374).

Another symbol with prenatal roots is that of the holy place or holy room, which recalls the uterus. Such a holy room cannot be simply chosen but must be "discovered." For this to happen, the "discoverer," to express it psychologically, must feel himself overcome by the reactivation of powerful prenatal emotions. In fact, mythology often makes use here of expressions from embryology. However, it is my opinion that these are not rational constructions but rather simple recognition of what has been repressed: "The Very Holy One made the world like an embryo. Just as the embryo begins to grow from the navel, so God made the world beginning with the navel and from there He extended Himself in all directions" (Eliade 1986, p. 434).

Often a tree of life stands in the middle of the holy room: "A tree or holy pillar which supports the world, a tree of life or a magic tree which gives immortality to those who eat of its fruit, because the tree incorporates absolute reality, the source of life and of holiness and is to be found at the centre of the world" (p. 437).

The memory of "such a holy room" or the yearning for such a place haunts mankind and leads to innumerable symbolizations and transformations (Plaut 1959). Eliade continues: "We understand that the homesickness for paradise is the yearning to be always and without any effort at the heart of the world, of reality and of the sacred. Put succinctly, in a completely natural way to leave what is human behind and achieve a state of divinity. A Christian would say the state before the Fall" (p. 441).

In a similar way, the myth of paradise also contains a certain projection of prenatal psychology. The prenatal Garden of Eden is threatened by the detachment of the fruit, which symbolizes the end of the prenatal period of growth and the fall from Heaven. The "evil" snake is another universal symbol, that of the negatively experienced umbilical cord. Around the time of birth, the cord no longer ensures an adequate supply of oxygen and, as one can speculate and as is reflected in many therapeutic regressions, is therefore sensed to be evil. In many myths the symbol of the snake appears in connection with transitions reflecting birth. During his uterine journey at night, the Egyptian Sun God is at first accompanied by a health-bringing snake. However, before dawn, which is pictured as a symbolic birth, he must confront the evil snake Apophis and kill it (Hornung 1984). The snake has thus two meanings. On the one hand, it is the protector of the tree and source of life, and, on the other, the evil dragon-snake that has to be killed to achieve the liberation of birth. Commensurate with the prenatal roots of this symbolism, snakes live in holes; the snake can then signify the uterus, the snake as swallower, as well as the umbilical cord, a violent birth is then expressed as the hero's fight in the dragon's throat.

Another symbol of the placenta, the eagle, may at first seem strange. However, this connection is suggested by a comparison of myths. The basis of this may be that the fetus experiences the placenta as hovering above him on the uterine sky. In any case, the eagle is a collective symbol that is used in a very similar way in all cultures and periods of history. The eagle and the tree of life are also often placed together and in their function can stand in for one another. Among the Jakuti, an eagle hatches the shamans out of an egg in a holy tree. Just as it is the Tree of Life in some myths, in others it is the eagle that supplies or is even identical with the elixir of life, the drink that guarantees immortality. Like the Tree of Life, the eagle is also considered to be a human ancestor (Sternberg 1930). In many myths, the eagle and snake appear together, just as the crown and the trunk of the tree of life symbolism are always directly connected. In the ancient Sumerian Ethana myth, it is said: "At that time, an eagle and a snake were alive. At first, they lived in peace and harmony with each other" (Egli 1982, p. 254). In many mythologies, there is a battle between the eagle and snake at the beginning of historical times. That is, psychologically speaking, the unity between the placenta and the umbilical cord breaks and positive and negative forces come into conflict. The report of the Ethana myth continues: "Then, however, enmity appeared between them and the eagle said to the snake: 'I will eat your offspring!'" (p. 254).

Other myths emphasize the harmony between the eagle and the snake. The Maya express the harmony of the cosmos in the symbol of a snake-bird, and in the Minoan culture the mother-goddess is sometimes depicted as a snake and sometimes as a bird.

An important theme in mythology is that of the end of the world, the final cosmic catastrophe, which from a prenatal psychology point of view gains its deep significance from the fetus's experience of the destruction of his prenatal world during birth. The well-known example is the Germanic idea of Ragnarök or cosmic conflagration, which is followed by a new creation. Fire is a frequent birth symbol that Frédérick Leboyer (1986) connects with the stimulation of the skin that occurs during birth.

The various Creation myths contain diverse pictures of the experiences of birth. These are used by a culture in its distinct cultural context to express its own identity. However, the description and interpretation of these myths lies outside the scope of this book. It can be concluded that the shaman, and all those descended from him who seek healing, strive to retrieve the sublime existence that they enjoyed in the prenatal world and that is made tangible for them in the symbols of the Water and the Tree of Life. Eliade (1986) writes:

> Immortality is difficult to attain. It is concentrated in the Tree of Life (or the Spring of Life) which is to be found in an inaccessible place at the end of the world, at the bottom of the ocean, in the land of darkness, on the top of the most high mountain or at the "centre." A monster (a snake) guards the tree and a man, who has reached the tree after considerable struggles, has then to fight the monster and to conquer it in order to be able to take possession of the fruit of immortality. [p. 333]

To strengthen his ego, the hero has thus to go through the dangers of his birth struggle once more.

It is interesting for the field of psychohistory that the Indo-Germanic deities are said to have developed out of the image of the eagle. With this as their prototype, the totemic origin of the idea of God is immediately revealed. The reference to the placenta is even clearer in the case of totem animals. In some Indian languages, placenta and totem are even described by the same word, *Nagual* (Brinton 1984). The totem thus expresses the continuity of the relationship to the placenta. The security that is experienced prenatally in the relationship to the placenta serves, in the symbolic form of the totem, in a creative way to articulate social structures. An individual finds himself to be in a similar mystical symbiosis with the group as he was with his placenta (Bächtold-Stäubli 1987a, Davidson 1985, Long 1963).

Through using totems, mankind was able to create cultural entities that were able to far outlive the hordes and groups driven together only by instinct. The transformation of tribal culture into high culture, the gradual mutation of structures still directly dependent on prenatal, totemic symbols into high cultures based on postnatal patterns can be followed in a fascinating way in the case of the Egyptian Pharaohs (Frankfort 1942). At first they were given totemic animal names. The same happened with the totem as with the placenta which can be symbolized as guardian spirit, animal, and brother. Out of the totem grew the symbolism of the Egyptian Ka. In the African tribe, the Kpell, the word *Kasen* is used to describe the totem. But it can also be translated as "birth thing" and thus explained as "that which is a person's back." That is almost the same as the meaning that the *Handbook of German Superstition* (Bächtold-Stäubli 1987c, p. 1038) gives for the Egyptian Ka. It is also possibly the same as the Nordic *Fylgji*, which has the meaning of "companion soul." These few suggestions are enough to show just how fruitful it could be for the psychology of culture to study the roots of experience in the prenatal stage of life.

BETWEEN HEAVEN AND HELL

It is quite plausible to connect the notion of Heaven as a place of bliss with a projection of good prenatal conditions. In fact, it is the experience of prenatal security that imparts the certainty that there is such a place where the blessed live. Ideas about Heaven blend here with ideas about paradise— the place where mankind comes from is also the place to which it returns. Etymologically, paradise has the meaning of "enclosure" or of "orchard" or "park" (Kluge 1967, p. 531).

Conversely, the mythological ideas of Hell are projective symbolizations of negative circumstances within the womb. And it is conspicuous that in the older myths Heaven and Hell are more or less indistinguishable from one another. The path to Hell leads through great hardships or is a fall into the abyss. Hell is often separated from the rest of world by water or a wall. Often it is imagined to be underground, in Mother Earth. Images of Hell became peculiarly extreme in Egypt and in the Christian culture.

The Egyptian images are nothing less than a collection of horrors representing perinatal crises: the dead have to walk on their heads, swallow their own excrement, can no longer move freely; the dead are tied and fettered, they are beheaded, butchered, beaten, killed, and cut down. Air to breathe is stolen from them or cut off. The threshold to Hell is a "watery, dark abyss which as the jaws of hell swallows sinners" (Hornung 1968, p. 172). The association with birth is also manifest in the fact that the Egyptian birth goddess is called "Mistress of the Slaughter." In early Egyptian culture it was assumed that Hell was in the body of a snake or in that of a goddess (Hermsen 1993, 1996).

In Christianity the entrance to Hell is also thought of as the jaws of a dragon or dog and is also expressed by the idea of *vagina dentata*. Perhaps in these images in which good and evil are so radically separated, the image of suffering in Hell is even more severe than it is in the Egyptian religion. The theme of burning, which is also contained in the idea of Purgatory, can, as has already been said, be associated with the extreme feelings of burning in the skin that occur during birth. Hell, however, is also described as extremely cold and the experience of temperature change at birth may be reflected in this.

SACRIFICE AS BIRTH

According to the information we now have, life in earlier cultures was determined in many and various ways by sacrificial rituals. For every human activity or every special event, the performance of a sacrifice could facilitate psychological processing. Put another way, in the early stages of culture, the individual felt so weak that only recourse to ritual execution bestowed sufficient stability for independent action. All self-determined concerns can trigger fear and feelings of guilt, and these feelings ultimately go back to the primal action of bringing one's self into the world. At the same time, being born involved sacrificing the original unity of mother and child. To this extent, then, autonomous action is always deeply fraught by the breach of a primal symbiosis, an original sin. It is these deep-reaching feelings that can be sorted out in the performance of sacrifices. The French ethnologists Henri Hubert and Marcel Mauss (1968) have shown that the process of sacrifice includes prenatal regression: "After a purifying bath, the victim is given newly made clothes which demonstrate that a new form of existence has begun for him. After various anointings, he is then clothed in the skin of a black antelope. That is the sacred moment in which a new being appears within him. He has become a fetus" (p. 20).

As a fetus, he then separates himself from the totemic, sacrificial animal whose placental significance has just been discussed above. The sacrifice of the animal victim reenacts an essential element of birth, the cutting of the umbilical cord, the very first sacrifice that made entry into the world possible. This sacrifice is at the same time self-sacrifice because it is the abandonment of the prenatal form of existence. The aim of the sacrifice is renewal by relating back to our origins and then making a new beginning. Eliade (1986) expressed it thus: "We have to be satisfied with the knowledge that with every sacrifice the Brahman repeats the cosmogonic act and that this coincidence of the 'mythical moment' with the 'present moment' signifies not only the destruction of profane time but also the lasting renewal of the world" (p. 91).

It is psychohistorically important that sacrificial rituals in India have been superseded by yoga techniques. This signifies an internalization of the rite of sacrifice. The asceticism of the yogi is a "sacrifice." Eliade (1985) writes: "We prefer to call this form of sacrifice 'internalisation of the ritual' because apart from inner prayer it involves a profound conformation of physiological functions with cosmic life. This homologisation of physiological organs and functions with cosmic realms and rhythms is a pan-Indian phenomenon" (p. 121).

This conformation symbolizes the prenatal state of life with its union of the fetus and mother. However, it is no longer symbolized in an external sacrificial ritual but in inner experience. The psychohistorical development of the West can be understood in the fact that the original sacrifice of the early high cultures was superseded by the sacrifice of Christ and the self-sacrifice of Christian suffering and of Christian moral conduct. Also here, symbolic sacrifice generates a link with a world beyond which itself symbolizes the projection of a good prenatal state.

This transition from sacrificial ritual that served renewal and psychological integration to the inner practices of the Yogi and the self-discipline of the Christian way of life represent stages of an expansion of consciousness and a more complete individuation. Increasing ego strength and decline of ritual, myth and fairy tale led to a shift in attitude to life in the direction of an increased sense of personal individuality, a shift that was ripened during the nineteenth century. Early experience, which until then had been projected into myth, ritual, and fairy tale, was increasingly rediscovered to be personal feelings and life history. This psychohistorical shift was expressed at the end of the nineteenth century in the German-speaking world in Freud's early psychoanalysis. The Oedipus myth was realized to be and psychologically named the oedipal conflict, a stage in biography. At first, however, only the reference to the father became explicit in Freud. The reference to the mother in the first part of the Oedipus myth, the prenatal trauma caused by the parental conflict and the perinatal trauma of exposure, was first explicitly formulated by Freud's students.

YOGA AND BIRTH

There is much support for the idea that yoga exercises essentially represent prenatal regression and trance, or rather the activation of states of fetal consciousness and the detachment and independence from the outer world. However, whereas shamanistic regression is completely dedicated to the purposes of healing and the resolution of social conflicts, the regression within yoga meditation totally serves individual development and detachment from bondage to

the world. Yoga ceremonies contain diverse symbols of
uterine regression; the parallels go so far that the yogi allows
himself to be buried alive in Mother Earth. He becomes
independent of the provision of external nourishment and
can more or less do without breathing. The regression is
evoked by what Eliade (1985) calls *embryonal breathing*: "The
purpose of this breathing is, according to Taoist sources, to
imitate the breathing of the fetus in the womb. It is said in
the foreword to the 'Tai-si K'eou Kioe,' that when one
returns to the foundation, one goes back to the origin, one
dispels age and returns to the state of a fetus" (p. 77).
Another aspect of the induction of regression is the yoga
positions. These can be interpreted as sophisticated reenactments of the pre- and perinatal expression (Crisan
1994).

For the embryo, the navel and umbilical cord are
central elements of existence—in yoga, meditation is induced by concentration on the navel. In tantric yoga, the
uterine regression can also be produced by making or gazing
at a mandala, that is, something on the visual-imaginative
level. Contemplation of a mandala leads through a belt of
fire, a door and labyrinth, symbols of birth, into an inner
paradise (Fischle 1982).

The symbolism of prenatal objects in Buddhist meditation is also interesting for prenatal psychology. The imaginative representation of the umbilical cord as the trunk of
the World Tree and the Axis of the World is apparently
universal. Eliade (1985) writes:

Characteristically in the Vedas, the mythic image of the
Brahman, of the Skambha, the cosmic pillars, *axis mundi*, is a
symbol the antiquity of which requires no further proof since
it is to be found among the hunters and herdsmen of Central

and Northern Asia as well as among the "primitive cultures" of Oceania, Africa and the Americas. . . . In other words, the Brahman is the ground which supports the world, at one and the same time World Axis and ontological foundation." [p. 124]

The internalization of the feeling of prenatal security is the root of the later self since the self is always based upon a residue of original, primal narcissism. Similar speculations on this subject are to be found in the Upanishads:

Being identified with the "axis" of the universe is to be found on another level in the spiritual "centre" of a person, the Atman. The one who recognises the Brahman in a person also recognises the highest being. And whoever recognises the highest being, recognises the Skambha. One sees the effort involved in comprehending the highest reality, the principle which cannot be formulated in words. Brahman as pillar of the universe is recognised as the support, the basis . . . but to know the Skambha means to possess the key to the cosmic secrets. It is the discovery of the "centre of the world" in the most profound depths of one's own being. This knowledge is a sacred force for it resolves the mystery of the universe and the mystery of the self. As is to be expected, the universal principle, the Brahman, is identified with the Brahmans." [Eliade 1985, p. 125]

The unification of the feeling of prenatal security with the spiritual security of the postnatal ego, which in the teachings of the Brahmans takes place on a more intellectual level, is realized in yoga more or less on the physical level. The exercises reproduce a prenatal unity.

OMNIPOTENCE AND THE DOWNFALL
OF THE RULER

Prenatal psychology is still completely speculative in the analysis of social processes. Nevertheless it can already be certified that sociocultural processes are determined in very important ways by the projection of pre- and perinatal experiences. It seems that social solidarity, which was inadequate among the hunters and gatherers, was achieved in the formation of large groups in early agricultural societies by collective and socially accepted projections of pre- and early postnatal images of the parents. This projection of feelings of prenatal security upon spiritual and secular leaders was an antidote to the elementary ignorance and fear experienced in an inhospitable world.

I understand that this emotional projection induced an alignment of will and a creative channeling of the group's energies. It was this that enabled the impressive technical, social, and cultic achievements of the early high cultures. Apparently, however, this then had the effect that the leaders in the early high cultures lived in a sort of psychotic state. They had to act as if they were immortal and omnipotent in order to maintain the projection of fetal omnipotence. Joseph Campbell writes: "The rulers of the Egyptian dynasties assumed that it was part of their temporal nature to be God, that is, they were insane. They were confirmed, brought up, flattered and encouraged in this belief by parents, priesthood, wives, counsellors and the people and everyone who also believed that they were god. That means that the whole of society was insane" (quoted in Wilber 1987, p. 139).

However, there was method in this madness. As already stated, the ruler symbolized prenatal omnipotence and reflected it to everyone so that in this way the social solidarity of such large groups that had come into existence artificially and their ability to produce technological and cultural innovations could be secured.

These associations might explain the peculiar and well-documented royal sacrifices that served to bring about renewal. Through ritual executions, symbolic of birth, the sacrifices were intended to secure reconnection with the origin and revitalization. The prenatal, symbiotic relationship between the king and his people also explains the peculiar and remarkable killings that took place at the same time as the death of the ruler (DeMause 1989a). The whole royal court that was directly connected with him accompanied him into the grave. It is testified that four thousand people were killed at the death of the Inca ruler, Huaryna Capac (Davies 1981).

The radical nature of the archaic warfare practiced in the early high cultures also becomes understandable within this framework of interpretation. The steady equilibrium based upon ideas of omnipotence is immediately thrown into question by any rival power and then swings over into rudimentary birth aggression. Extreme forms of warfare were developed in the early city-states dependent on agriculture. These city-states formed, as in the case of Egypt, a self-sufficient cosmos. As described above, their solidarity was maintained through prenatal symbolism. The walled city is itself a picture of uterine security which is then represented once more in the sacred buildings in the city center. Trapped in the illusion of fetal omnipotence as they were, these political entities were unable to resolve conflicts. The Egyptian State of the Old Kingdom is said to have been unable to make contracts with other states. This is because the existence of a state, somehow of equal standing as itself, lay beyond the horizon envisaged in the symbolism of fetal omnipotence.

Any questioning of omnipotence signifies the end of prenatal security, the world of fetal projection and leads to the struggle of birth. Only a victory can restore the early condition. Here as an example is a war report from Sumer:

> Sargon, King of Agade, conquered the city of Uruk and demolished its walls. He fought with the people of Uruk and wiped them out. He also fought against Lugal-Zaggisi, King of Uruk, took him prisoner and led him in chains through the door of Enlil. Sargon of Agade fought with the man from Ur and conquered him. He conquered the city and demolished its walls. [Wilber 1987, p. 186]

The fetal omnipotence of King Sargon had been thrown into question by the existence of the more or less equally powerful King of Uruk. He had to conquer him or the whole system would have to change.

Now one can see the history of culture as being determined in its essentials by the attempt on the one hand to secure social solidarity by the suggestion of prenatal security and at the same time to make the operative structures within this framework gradually more rational and flexible. Even until the twentieth century, the solidarity of national and multinational groups was maintained by symbolizations of primal security that appear to us today as peculiarly childish, for example, the divine right of kings or later the claims to omnipotence of various ideologies. In the course of historical development, however, primitive projections and their confirmation in events of collective, ritual trance, such as we see in the old high cultures, were retracted. This is the expression of increasing social and technological skill and the personal affirmation that can be achieved through true mastery of reality. This corresponds well to a transformation in personal identity, which was expressed psychohistorically at the turn of the nineteenth century. It became possible to face personal emotions and individual development with its "dying and becoming" with an increased inner freedom and without then feeling the necessity to act them out destructively.

One can also interpret the development suggested here as follows: the early cultures with their social creation of the figure of the ruler started something like what we understand to be personal development. This is because the ruler exemplified an independence of will that was then reflected back and internalized. If in the beginning only Osiris was the Pharaoh, in the end all Egyptians were Osiris. Whereas in the beginning only the ruler participated in immortality, with the Christian faith everyone could lay claim to an immortal soul and our ideas about individualism are based on this. It seems to me that these are all aspects of mankind constituting itself in culture through the creative use of the primal experience of the two worlds.

BATTLE

In the history of culture, we can recognize processes of initiation through *regressus ad uterum*, through sacrifice, and also through battle. Battle as a method of individual development has become known to us especially from American Indian culture; it is unusual to point out the perinatal association. It is, however, very tangible in the early ritual forms of battle. Gladiatorial contests have their roots in the ritual fighting that took place at funerals (Grant 1982). If dying is experienced as a symbolic return to the mother, then of necessity at the same time the struggle of birth must also be repeated. It might thus be possible to understand why people in ancient Rome frequently specified in their wills that a gladiatorial duel had to take place at their funerals. Historically speaking, the main reason for such battles was also the commemoration of the deceased. When the perinatal associations are under consideration, the various forms of single combat, such as fighting with wild animals or with nets, can be understood as reenactments of frightful and aggressive birth struggles. Fighting with a wild animal or being caught in a net can in a dream symbolize the struggle of birth. The elaboration of single combat into a mass spectacle only began in the third century before Christ.

The ritual aspect of fighting also still survived in the Roman custom of the "Devotio" (Gehrts 1967). By that is meant that in order to gain victory over the enemy, one of the two Roman generals who together led the Army consecrated himself to the Underworld. Fully armed, he would fall into the hands of the enemy and allow himself to be killed. This expiatory sacrifice guaranteed victory for the other general. To "deliver the glory of victory" a cleansing sacrifice was required. Psychologically it can be said that birth is only possible by going through death. This perinatal background is alive in many ideas of war. Victory is achieved by experiencing death in the slaughter. After a victory, the Roman general was allowed to celebrate with a festive procession through the Arch of Triumph, a symbol of birth.

Initiatory fighting gains its meaning from the significance of the struggle of birth, which causes individuation and change. In the Greek Olympic competitions the initiatory aspect is also quite obvious. They assisted the personal development of the competitors. The prize was the laurel wreath, a branch of the Tree of Life. The perinatal symbolism active within the experience of fighting is especially apparent at the onset of war. The American psychohistorian Lloyd DeMause (1989a, b), has drawn attention to this. War is to some extent the solution to a conflict or crisis that is experienced as perinatal constriction. Words such as *pushed, crushed,* and *strangled,* which express sensations that occur during birth, have a central place in declarations of war. Thus, Kaiser Wilhelm said, as he pronounced the beginning of the First World War, that he felt "choked" because suddenly "a net has been thrown over our heads." Hitler explained that he went to war in order to resolve Germany's *Lebensraum-Frage.* Similarly, American declarations from the beginning of the Civil War until Vietnam contain phrases such as "Independence is fighting for its existence," "sinking into the abyss," and the impossibility of "seeing light at the end of the tunnel" (DeMause 1979b, p. 59). As Klaus Theweleit in his *Male Fantasies* (1977) has shown, such perinatal symbolism is also central to the experience of fascist men. Their central fantasy is of "self-negation" (German: *selbstverschmelzung*) in battle, "separation from the rotting, capsizing world (female swamp)," and "rebirth and ascent."

From the perspective of these ideas, one can see war as the expression of the collective, secularized initiation of large groups, symbolic of birth and containing all the elements of initiatory combat. I have described above how large groups even until today are held together in unseen ways by fantasies of fetal security that are connected with certain cultural ideals. When two such groups confront one another, the fantasy of fetal omnipotence collapses, and from the point of view of depth psychology the only remaining solution is a birth struggle that is then realized in war. One can only reach freedom and a new world through the "abyss of slaughter."

Of course, the same can happen when the foundations of a culture are annulled by technical or social innovation and the fantasies of omnipotence that are connected to them begin to collapse. Here the only thing from early experience that helps to achieve a new and stable condition is the struggle of birth. A glimmer of hope in our times can be seen in the fact that through retracting archaic projections, individuals and groups have become more able to cope with conflict and transformation. That is, to resolve collective conflicts, the dynamics of change are managed in inner births and in symbolic activities within society instead of in real massacres (DeMause 1996, Wasdell 1991a, b, 1993, 1995).

Above all else, the primal therapy pioneered by Arthur Janov has shown with what intensity perinatal, primal pain is present within every one of us. Every real change, precisely because our deep experience conceives of it as a repetition of birth, can activate this primal pain. As a result, processes of social change that had become critical, such as revolutions, could until now as a rule not progress without dramatic events, symbolic of birth. The world within the mother in which the fetus was previously hidden and which he survived has got to die so that a new one can be born. These are not abstract constructs but stem from the elementary, personal experiences of the events of birth (DeMause 1991, 1996, Grof 1983, Janus 1995a, Wasdell 1993).

Because research into prenatal relationships has not been carried out, the extent to which social dependence behavior has prenatal roots seems to me to be still completely uncertain. When it does become clear, phenomena of human exploitation such as slavery may become more understandable.

IMAGES OF PRIMAL EXPERIENCE

Pre- and perinatal experiences have always influenced art in a disguised way, simply because life in the womb and birth are fundamental human experiences (Irving 1989). Thus the Danish Arts scholar Johannes Fabricius (1991), has been able by careful interpretation to show just how latent pre- and perinatal symbols can be found in classical works of art. Rembrandt's 1653 painting, *Ganymede and the Eagle*, can briefly illustrate this. Zeus has fallen in love with Ganymede and kidnaps the youth in the form of an eagle. Fabricius interprets this painting in which the eagle Ganymede is rising up into the sky as follows:

> For many reasons, the way in which Rembrandt has painted this saga is puzzling. Firstly, he painted the youth Ganymede as a small child with a contorted body. Furthermore, Ganymede's face is marked by an intense emotion of traumatic fear and he is urinating because of shock. The result is the transformation of the gods' cupbearer into a screaming infant with repulsively twisted face and body. All art historians are agreed that Rembrandt has portrayed a Ganymede that Zeus would never have chosen.
>
> Ganymede's hoisted tunic looks like the large and small lips of the vulva. The lower part of a baby's body is falling out of this and he is urinating because of fear during birth. . . .
>
> The head of the child is inside an image of a projected uterus. The black, feathered abdomen of the bird represents the womb against the cavelike walls of which the child is

pressing his right hand. The wavering tassel inside can be interpreted to be the umbilical cord." [p. 72]

The association, however, was more explicitly expressed only in our century (Janus 1994). The direct portrayal of regressive, biographical details has been one of the major impulses within modern art. Klee (1975), for example, says that "our worlds have been opened" (p. 58). By this he means the "realm of the unborn" to which "children, the insane and primitive peoples" (p. 58) have perhaps an even more direct contact. The direct portrayal of the unconscious, the core of which consists of pre- and perinatal experience, is an important part of the surrealists' intention. I would like to illustrate this with the example of Salvador Dalí who based much of his art directly upon pre- and perinatal experience.

It is certain that Dalí's strong interest in his prenatal life was influenced by the exceptional circumstances of his conception and birth. He said of himself that actually he did not really exist because he was conceived as a substitute for an older brother of his who had died. His biographer, Meryle Secrest (1987), writes:

Apparently he (Dalí) already became aware in his very early years that he was not loved for who he was. When he looked into the eyes of his mother, he did not see his own reflection but that of a ghost. . . . His cousin said: "His parents made comparisons every day between the two. She gave him the same clothes and the same toys. She treated him as if he were the other and Dalí got the impression that he did not really exist." Dalí said that his father was pushed into despair because "He saw my double just as much as he saw me myself. For him, I was only half myself, one half too much. My soul was worn down by worry and rage. Under this laser beam which permanently searched for someone else who no longer existed. And I had in my soul a bleeding wound which my father cold, heartless, without any consideration for my tormented emotions, continually opened with a love that struck me like a cudgel." [p. 31]

We know from psychotherapy that, in cases where early relationships are so broken, the very earliest experiences remain accessible to consciousness. Dalí (1973) describes this aspect of himself: "My parents' despair [due to the loss of the brother] was only soothed by my birth but every cell of their body had sucked itself full of their grief. My fetus swam in a hellish placenta. I have never been able to get rid of this affliction" (p. 10).

He describes (1984) his intrauterine memories as follows:

The intrauterine paradise was the colour of hell, that is, red, orange, yellow, bluish, the colour of flames, of fire. Above all else, it was warm, immobile, soft, symmetrical, duplex and sticky. Already even then, all pleasure and enchantment was located in eyes and the most wonderful, the most eye-catching imagination was that of two eggs frying in a pan, but without the pan. Probably every confusion, every emotion can be traced back to the fact that for the rest of my life since then I perceive under the influence of this abiding, hallucinatory image. [1984, p. 42]

It is a well-known game among children to press on the eyeballs in order to see rings of color that are then sometimes called angels. As Dalí seems to suggest, the child is thereby trying to reconstruct visual memories from the embryonal period. The artist describes very vividly how in a

complicated ceremony he attempted every evening to trans-
port himself back into a prenatal state.

He wrote the following about the method he used to
produce prenatal images within himself:

> I go down on all fours so that my knees and my hands are
> touching. Then I allow my head to hang down under its own
> weight and to swing like a pendulum so that lots of blood
> runs into it. I do this exercise until a pleasurable dizziness sets
> in. Without having to shut my eyes, I see phosphorescent
> rings emerging out of the pitch black darkness[1] in which the
> celebrated fried eggs without the frying pan begin to form.
> [1984, p. 47]

The symbiosis with Gala (his wife) also served Dalí as a
"feeler" to bring him in touch with the prenatal beyond.
Many pictures show how Gala, clearly in some sort of a
trance, mutates into fetal symbolism—a path into a forest, a
fantastic building, everything in an atmosphere of floating
and prenatal emotion.

I have discussed and quoted Dalí extensively because his
paintings are so well known and because many readers will
be able to relate to them. In some paintings the fetal
symbolism is very clear. In *The Return of Christ*, a human with
umbilical-like strands is connected to the figure of a dragon,
symbolizing the placenta. Threads and ropes, symbols of the
umbilical cord, hanging down from the sky regularly appear
in his paintings.

The modern awareness of early personal experiences is
expressed in Dalí's art in a very extreme form. On the one
hand, he tries to a certain extent to unload his early,

---

1. Darker than real darkness in which things can still be seen.

regressive fears onto others, and, on the other, he wants to bring the viewers into contact with their own personal experiences. He developed this way of discharging his own fears in his youth in what he called his "paranoia-critical method." By seeing clearly, he used all his own contradictions to help others to feel the fears and ecstasy within their own life so that this would gradually become as real and essential as his own. It can also be expressed as follows: from within his own deeply felt rootlessness (German: *Heimatlosigkeit*), he developed increasingly more radical ways of being noticed by others. The huge success of Salvador Dalí's art testifies to how widespread are the sorts of experience that he addressed and indicated.

Pre- and perinatal associations are even more "physically" expressed and encountered in the performance art of the 1970s and 1980s. Joseph Beuys's 1974 performance, "Coyote," has been interpreted by the psychoanalyst Hartmut Kraft (1991) as a shamanistic regression to the womb and rebirth. In this performance, Beuys was wrapped in felt and spent eight days in a cage with a coyote. The placenta and umbilical symbols in the work of Joseph Beuys were recently interpreted by the German physician and psychotherapist Dieter Arnold (1996). Peter Gilles's performances (Kraft 1991) and the performance artists in Vienna also make an impact by using pre- and perinatal symbolism. (Meifert 1990, Meifert and Meifert 1991).

THE CONTINUUM OF SOUND

Music and sounds have always been able to lift people above their everyday drudgery. Hearing is the sense that, alongside those of balance and movement, is responsible from the middle of the pregnancy onward for the relationship of the fetus to the mother and the outside world. Furthermore, it links up directly with postnatal auditory experience. Everything that was heard before birth is recognized after birth and thus forms a bridge between the two worlds. As is expressed in Mozart's *Magic Flute*, this tonal bond straddles the dangers of birth. Tamino and Pamina gain the strength necessary for the initiation, symbolic of birth, from music. Music gives them the power to endure the anxieties connected with real individuation.

According to the French doctor and hearing specialist Alfred Tomatis, the beginning of our experience of sound occurs as we hear the noises made by the ears themselves as they develop, the movements of the cells and the lymph, and the vibrations of the hair cells. This is the "unhearable sound" that mystics seek in their meditation, the "sound of life" as Tomatis (1987 p. 176) calls it.

Whether that is so or not, it is the sounds of the maternal heartbeat, of the mother's body, and of her voice that mark the baby's auditory experiences before birth. It is conceivable that this fundamental, primal experience resounds in the rhythms, movements, and singing voices of our postnatal music and dance. Music has always had the power to enchant us and to rouse other states of consciousness and early experience within us (Parncutt 1993, Rotter 1985).

The variety of auditory experiences before birth is very easy to underestimate. The conductor Boris Brott tells the following story:

> "It may sound strange but music was already a part of me before my birth. . . . As a young man, I was astounded by my unusual ability to play certain pieces without the score. As I

conducted a piece for the first time, the cello part suddenly caught my attention and I knew how the piece continued even before I turned the page. One day I mentioned it to my mother who is a professional cellist. I thought it would astonish her that it was always the cello part which stood so clearly before my eyes. She was amazed. But then, as she heard which pieces of music were involved, the mystery was unravelled. All the pieces which I knew without the score were the ones which she had played during the time she was pregnant with me." [quoted in Verny and Kelly 1983, p. 16]

It is tempting to explain the frequently unbelievable ability of some people to grasp complex musical structures as being based on prenatal auditory experience. The continuity of auditory experience is ordained to be a channel for initiatory experience, as happens during all feasts.

The primal therapist Peter Orban (1980) has described the regressive power of music in a therapeutic experience:

I had the opportunity of participating in a five-day marathon with the American therapist, Dan Miller, in which he activated the birth experiences of between 6 and 14 participants only with the use of relaxation exercises and music by Paul Horn ("Inside") that is, without words. The participants were transported literally into the fetal situation, that is, into their "within" only through the power of the music—bizarre flute music played "within" the Taj Mahal Tomb." [p. 6]

One of Arthur Janov's patients reported:

"Actually twice during my therapy, I experienced something peculiar. Only on the second occasion did I realise that a certain piece of music had brought me back to my birth feelings. This special music contains deep bass tones (some-

thing like the music of Quincy Jones). It produce a certain
feeling of hopefulness in me (We'll make it, baby!) I felt the
dark bass, my head lifted up (chin in the air), pressed
backwards against my neck and within seconds I had fallen
onto the bed and was a fetus making rhythmic movements
(working), fighting for the way I wanted to go. I assume that
music is partly—as are words—a symbolic description of
birth emotions." [Janov 1974, p. 87]

In a similar way, classical music and rock and pop music
can activate "oceanic feelings," the experience of being one
with the music and in communion with the universe. Only it
seems to happen in modern pop music more directly. The
beat leads immediately to an inner resonance with the
primal experience of the maternal heartbeat and of the fetal
self.

We know from therapy that music of the various youth
cultures can have a stabilizing effect during the critical years
of puberty. Resonance with primal experience can give a
person a feeling of continuity within his or her identity:
"Young people believe that they then know and feel 'where
they are heading.' The beat is thus like a scaffolding, a
second skeleton, an artificial limb and in addition supports
continuity within personal identity by means of narcissistic
skin sensations" (Hoffmann 1988, p. 965).

The social scientist Carla Mureck (1990) has described
the initiatory aspects of contemporary "destroyed music"
(dissonant modern music) with much insight:

If one allows these noises to have an effect, it is as if the small,
pitching boat of the fragile self had fallen into the roaring
pandemonium of a hurricane, as Poe described it. It is as if
one has been shot into a black hole in which it is said that

space and time are reversed and that it is the suction out of which our planets were born and into which we will return and perish. . . . It is the music of dreaming, a music like being outside of the universe, "Stalker music," which accompanies us into forbidden zones. On the one hand, the clash of archaic-simple sounds and on the other, machine and industrial noises . . . confront the world of natural man and of the child with the adult world of work and war. [p. 128]

The presence of sound patterns from the mother's voice in the cries of premature babies shows just how deeply prenatal hearing is interwoven with the making of noises and of hearing after birth. As early as 1966 in a pioneer study, the psychotherapist Günter Clauser (1971) demonstrated the influence of prenatal auditory experiences on the later development of language. The evidence concerning the collective experience of language before birth may be the reason modern nations constitute themselves around language as the element that binds the community.

THE HUMAN EXPERIENCE OF BEING THROWN INTO THE WORLD

Psychoanalysis sees that the important mythical personages and images documenting the development of human awareness have been raised to a new level of rationality in philosophy and have once more received a new form there. The original waters of myth becomes Thales's water, the origin of all things. The womb as origin is even preserved within more abstract concepts of being. Whereas a myth is still a direct and emotionally charged image of original experience, philosophy signifies on the contrary an enlightenment in which the mythic projection is revealed. At the same time, however, it creates a new myth, the belief in the omnipotence of reason, which Plato imagined as a symbolic realm of ideas located before birth. According to Plato, it was necessary to regain this comprehensive cognizance preceding earthly existence. Ultimately, this amounts to the archaic idea of perfection that is to be achieved by connecting prenatal with postnatal existence. On the level of myth, this perfection is gained by a journey to the underworld, which makes primal knowledge accessible (Janus 1990b).

In his famous analogy of the cave, Plato is, however, concerned to show just how few achieve this primal connection and attain perfection. Many remain trapped in the existential changeover that took place in the critical moments of their birth. A psychological birth that embraces both areas of their life does not take place. Many examples here make it possible to show how pre- and perinatal experience is processed in philosophical systems. However, I will continue the theme developed in our consideration of Dalí, namely, that questions about the significance of birth have become especially evident in the twentieth century. This is so in the work of Martin Heidegger.

One of the central concepts in *Being and Time* (1986) is that of *Geworfenheit*, that is "having-been-whelpedness," which names the fact of our having been born with a word from Heidegger's family background in farming. A person's "having-been-whelpedness" is always connected with his having fallen (*Verfallenheit*) into the world. In one place, he writes quite explicitly: "Factual being exists by birth and it also dies already at birth because *Seins zum Tode*—to exist is to die" (p. 374). This concept of *Seins zum Tode*, however, only hides the central problem of our having been born

(Ger. *Gebürtigkeit*). The subject that is exhaustively treated in Heidegger's philosophy is that of *Seins zum Tode*. This can be understood psychologically as an expression of the fear of birth. The same is true of *Hineingehaltensein ins Nichts* or "being held in nothingness." Just as Freud saw that birth fear determines basic human emotions, one of Heidegger's headings is "the basic emotion of fear as an excellent revelation of being" (p. 184).

Heidegger seems not to have assumed that there is experience of birth: "The fallenness (Ger. *Verfallenheit*) of existence must therefore not be understood as a fall out of a purer and higher 'primal state.' Not only have we no existential experience of such but also ontologically no possibility and guide to interpretation" (p. 176). As a result, he is also unable to think of the experience of death that so concerned him or the experience of one's own mortality in the context of our original birth experience. In answer to this, the philosopher Thomas Macho (1989) has tried to uncover the latent theme of birth that is hidden behind the analysis of death in Heidegger's thought in order to make a philosophy of our having-been-born-ness (Ger. *Geburtlichkeit*) possible. The philosophical thought of Peter Sloterdijk's aims in the same direction. It deals with the fact that birth has been forgotten by philosophy and attempts to comprehend human having-been-born-ness (*Geburtlichkeit*) in a philosophical way. He is the first philosopher to consider the prenatal dimension in man on a philosophical level and appreciate the psychoanalysts Rank and Graber as great humanistic pioneers (1993). The possibility of a female-oriented philosophy by recognizing the existential dimension of prenatal psychology is the subject of the Austrian philosopher Astrid Meyer-Schubert (1993).

ROBINSON CRUSOE'S INITIATION—
REBIRTH THROUGH POETRY

The theme of existence in the womb and birth appears in literature in various forms: as direct memory, as poetry, as a story line that follows the shaman's journey with its central elements of regression to the womb and rebirth, or as the motif of initiatory maturation found within a complete work.

An example of a memory of the earliest phases of life within a poem is the text found in Stifter's (1959) work which has already been quoted (p. 27). A structure reflecting birth in poetry, a projection onto the cosmos, is provided by Goethe's poem "Reunited" from the "West-Eastern Divan":

> When the world in deep conception
> Lay in God's eternal breast
> He so ordered its inception
> With sublime creative zest,
> And the word: "Become!" was spoken;
> With resounding painful shout
> Then the One, by power broken,
> To reality thrust out.
>
> Light appeared! immediately
> See the darkness parting shy,
> Elements each separately
> From each other further fly.
> Swift, in fierce wild dreaming legions,
> Each leapt out to distance bound,
> Rigid, through unmeasured regions,
> With no yearning, with no sound.
>
> God was first alone that morrow,
> All was silent, still, forlorn:

Then to love and comfort sorrow
He created red of dawn;
Colours through the gloom vibrated,
Harmonies resolving pain,
All that first was alienated
Now once more could love again.

All belonging seeks its pleasure,
Swift towards itself returns;
And to life which has no measure
All that sees, all feeling turns:
Seizing, snatching, all unheeded
If it only grips and holds!
[*Goethes Werke*, vol. II 1967, p. 83ff]

In his commentary, Erich Trunz (1967) writes: "Goethe had got used to seeing himself in relation to the cosmos and that was especially true for important moments of life. A depiction of the creation of the world is given here. . . . The world is imperfect because it is divided. . . . Love leads what has been separated together again" (p. 606).

Goethe had this to say about his birth: "As a result of ineptitude on the part of the midwife, I was born dead and they only managed that I saw the light of day after much trouble" (*Goethes Werke*, vol. IX 1967, p. 10).

In Goethe's *Poetry and Truth*, every aspect of the theme of birth is disguised in a sort of philosophical-mystical speculation in which the process of Creation is controlled by Lucifer and threatens to "annihilate itself in perpetual concentration." This standstill during birth is overcome by the Elohim, merciful beings, so that resurrection can follow death and so that at the end of this section, he can formulate the worldly wisdom of the possibility of unending individuation, self-transcendence and renewal: "That we are on one side forced to create ourselves and on the other that we must not forget at regular intervals to empty ourselves (Ger. *entselbstigen*)" (vol. XI, p. 353).

Symbolic regression in a place representing the womb and processes of return and denouement symbolic of birth are patterns of action that are seminal in literature. The theme is so comprehensive that there is not enough room here to deal with it adequately.

Alfred Kubin's 1909 novel *The Other Side* can be mentioned here as an example containing very little camouflage. Kubin created the story around the experience of a psychotic journey to regions within himself that occurred after a suicide attempt at his mother's grave.

Theodor Storm's (1982) *Regentrude* is an especially good example of the fact that coming to terms with fear of regression is a prerequisite of sexual maturity. Irmgard Roebling (1985) summarized it as follows:

> On the one hand, in a motif which is related in great detail, the journey of birth seems to have been reversed in the frightful departure of the two lovers through a small, spiral path into the inside of the earth. The pair reach a uterus-like building. When they unlock a spring, the place transforms itself into a damp, fragrant paradise full of flowers. [p. 85]

In the ballad "The Diver," Friedrich Schiller (1982) conceived of a journey to the depths with a comparable initiatory symbolism. The womb symbolism is very clear:

> And black out of the white foam
> A gaping slit opened downwards,

Bottomless, as if it led to hell,
And impetuous one sees the surging waves
Pulled down into the whirling crater. [p. 368]

In modern times, one of the most well-known stories involving an initiation is that of *Robinson Crusoe* (1719), which presents the cultural ideal of the modern *Homo faber* in the symbols of an adventure journey and transposition to another world. Irmgard Roebling (1990) has discerned the womb symbolism in the all-embracing and generous sea and the pelvis-like, enclosing cliffs of Crusoe's story. One can actually say that since the beginning of modern times a major part of the needs of young people for a fresh start during puberty has been satisfied by reading stories about initiation like that of Robinson Crusoe. A new version of the same thing is Michael Ende's *The Unending Story*, which involves many images of regression to the womb and a whole array of rebirth symbols and thus reflects the contemporary cultural ideal of pondering upon fantasy and emotion.

An example of how individuation is unsuccessful because of a birth that was too difficult is contained in Patrick Süskind's bestseller, *Perfume* (1985). Born enveloped by the smell of fish and left alone by his mother, the hero of the novel whose whole life is determined by the events of his birth tries of offset the trauma of the stench at his birth by becoming a scent specialist, the method of overcompensation as described by Alfred Adler. He then tries in a sort of Jungian womb regression inside a cave to overcome the circumstances of his traumatic birth. The perennial "usual stenches" are extinguished but a real recovery is unsuccessful. The criminal remedy, a murder, a further attempt to overcome the primal trauma is intrinsically doomed. Already "without rest" within the womb, he is also unable to find it in the world.

As Oskar Sahlberg (1986) has done in the case of Gottfried Benn, the motif of regression and rebirth can also be found within the whole progression of a literary work. Benn has again and again extolled the modern forms of "self-denial" (Ger. *Entselbstung*): "Ah, never enough of this experience: . . . Ah, continually in this fire, in the realm of the placental rooms, in the first stages of the ocean, the primal face: inclinations to regress, dissolution of the self!" (p. 2). In another place, Benn writes: "Art was always birth" (p. 3). Sahlberg shows by using the social psychological concepts of Germany's Third Reich, how the process of individuation in Benn ended disastrously. The connection between initiatory processes of individuation and poetic work can, as in the case of Benn, be clearly seen in many other poets.

The little known or discussed significance of the theme of birth in the literature and philosophy of the twentieth century can be shown graphically in the work of Samuel Beckett, who made the connection between pre- and peri-natal traumatization and the paradigm of his life's work, that of imperfect birth.

Together with his analyst, Bion, Beckett attended a lecture given by Jung in which he spoke about a female patient who was not born properly. Beckett's biographer, Deirdre Bair (1978) summarizes Beckett's experience: "Beckett found in Jung's words a key to the understanding of his relationship to his mother. If he was not perfectly born, if he had true prenatal memories and remembered his birth as painful, it seemed to him only logical that this ill-fated and defective, first happening in life had led to the unsatisfactory and imperfect development of his personality" (p. 209).

Because of its special significance, the encounter with Jung and its poetic portrayal in "Everything Which Falls" (1976) is quoted in detail. Here, a certain Mrs. Rooney attends a lecture by one of the modern doctors for "spiritual misery" which deeply impresses her;

> I remember how he told us the story of a young girl who was in her own way very peculiar and unhappy and how he treated her for years without success. Ultimately, he was forced to give up. He said that there was nothing wrong with her. The only thing the matter was, as far as he could find out, that she was dying away. And shortly after he had washed his hands in innocence, she did actually die. . . . What he said and the way in which he said it, has haunted me ever since. . . . When he was finished with this girl, he stood completely still for quite a while, easily two minutes, staring at the lectern. Then suddenly he lifted up his head and shouted as if he had just received a revelation: she had never been born properly! That's it, that is what was the matter with her. [p. 282ff]

Bair has even put forward the idea that it was Jung's lecture that triggered the mechanism behind Beckett's productivity.

However that may be, the image of the frustrated birth is a central point of reference in Beckett's work so that this thought is expressed, for example, in a central place in *Waiting for Godot*. Pozzo says before his departure: "One day we will be born, one day we die, on the same day, at the same moment. Is that not enough for you. They give birth astride the grave, the day lights up for a moment and then once again it is night" (p. 94). And Vladimir, another central character of the piece, repeats the same thought at the end in a slightly changed form. Through the impaired birth, the birth attendant becomes a grave digger: "Astride the grave and a difficult birth. Out of the depths of the pit, the grave digger as in a dream applies the forceps" (p. 96).

In addition to death, birth can also be expressed in the image of slaughter. Alfred Simon (1988) summarizes here: "Slaughter is always already present. Things are so. Birth is a slaughter, the first slaughter, one which makes it as equally impossible to live as to die" (p. 124). Further images for a tragic birth are those of falling and of expulsion:

> The birth of Hanswurst proceeded violently. We saw him falling down the outside staircase head first until he remained laying on the pavement. While the door locked itself again, his hat (thrown by invisible hands) flew through the air to him. Hanswurst was born with his hat on. Every hat . . . is for him a fetal bonnet. Birth is expulsion from the womb and every expulsion makes the outcast relive the mimodram of his birth in symbols once more. In reality, one is not born but rather thrown into the world. A second birth is required. One wants to be born in order at last to be able to die. The question of this second birth has remained unresolved and remains so until Beckett's last work. "Arriving in the world without being born," that is the key to slaughtering. [p. 124]

Beckett's significance in the history of thought is that his paradigm of the impeded birth coincided with the search for a new understanding of human existence in a world without myths and without God. In such a world in which a person is not welcomed into society by images institutionalized from the imagination of previous generations of parents, true arrival is very difficult to imagine:

> Thus Beckett's Nothing illustrates in his way the impossibility of recovering from the death of God. . . . The silly game

played by Beckett's clowns essentially consists of allowing the "gasping of those condemned to life" to be heard. . . . Beckett's clowns are the remnant of religious people which has not yet come to terms with the new order of things and which is now dying in endless, absurd convulsion. [p. 116]

Beckett's defective birth is curiously enough thoroughly comparable with the "not-having-been-born-completely" that Klaus Theweleit (1977) has discerned as the National Socialists' central problem. However, in the case of National Socialism it was more the death of the Kaiser, the death of the patriarchal, secular authority, that was unbearable and was to be overcome in a destructive way in the National Socialist rebirth ritual of war. Thus, one can speculate that something of the central, fascist problem of not having been born (Ger. *Ungeborenseins*), the failure to become an individual (Ger. *Unindividuiertheit*), and destructive-regressive yearning are expressed in the so-called theater of the absurd inspired by Beckett with its excess of birth symbolism. However, the dismissive category of the "absurd" also suggests how far we are from a true awareness of the crucial area of early experience.

It seems to me there are good reasons one can say that mediation between the prenatal and preverbal stage of life and later forms of socialization is one central concern of human culture. It is possible to understand Nietzsche's statement about the death of God as meaning that the way of cushioning postnatal, existential insecurity by institutionalized images of an omnipotent father is no longer possible, and that we find ourselves in a period of transition, searching for new forms of mediation in which psychotherapy has an increasingly significant role to play. Sloterdijk (1986) has

written something quite flippant but thoroughly true about
this:

> Psychotherapy has to do with people who suffer because they
> have to come to terms with their having fallen out the womb
> into late capitalism. And one has the feeling that this distance
> was too much. . . . This experience of the harshness of
> existence has influenced human life in the high cultures for
> at least three to four thousand years. The historical answer to
> this misunderstanding has been the high religions. . . . The
> disadvantage of having been born which all psychotherapy
> has to deal with stems from our discomfort in Reality, the "a
> priori oblique presentation" of our life to a social order which
> is obviously not the order which human life with its needs was
> prepared for. [p. 257]

In any case, *Waiting for Godot* or a "Führer" is no longer
an up-to-date solution. Beckett makes this clear by ridiculing
waiting for a God, using the English word *God* with the
French diminutive ending *-ot* (as in Jean/Jeannot).

In Goethe's poem "Blessed Longing" the paradigm of
birth is concisely formulated. Many thoughts about love and
initiation and death and rebirth are concentrated within it:

> Tell it no one, only sages,
> For the crowd derides such learning:
> Life I praise through all the ages
> Which for death in flames is yearning.
>
> Cooled in love-nights' animation,
> Which begat you, where you mated,
> You are seized by strange sensation,
> By still candlelight elated.

No more you are held in capture
Darkly over-shadowed waiting,
You anew are torn by rapture
Upwards to a higher mating.

From no weight of distance tiring
You're in spellbound flight held fast,
And you are, the light desiring,
Moth, in fire consumed at last.

Till by this you be possessed:—
Die and have new birth!
You are just a sombre guest
On the darkened earth.

10

The Fourth World of Mankind

We are at the end of an adventurous journey through the diverse manifestations in which our prenatal and birth experience continue to influence us. It should have become clear that these experiences and influences from the past are an intimate part of us. They are very deeply connected to our inner life. A description and consideration from only one perspective could never be comprehensive. Only a creative exploration of the conditions and long-term effects of the first phases of human life from various standpoints can throw light on its biographical significance. Our understanding of ourselves becomes more complete and, in the truest sense of the word, more human when we realize that our prenatal existence is a fourth world alongside the other three phases of human life, namely, childhood, adulthood, and old age.

It is a tragic aspect of the cultural development of our civilization in the last hundred years that our social reality, depending on our cultural point of view, is always in danger of disintegration. It is possible that the recognition of our prenatal existence will help us to gain a deeper awareness of the unity of the world at a new level of life, as it was in the Middle Ages, projected in the belief that we are all God's children. What Heidegger calls "forgetfulness of existence" (Ger. *Seinsvergessenheit*) in his philosophy appears in psychology as forgetting our prenatal origin. A deeper internalization of this dimension of our life could lead to a greater completeness of human existence. Our welfare does not lie in the projection of prenatal security. This is always in danger of bringing our life out of balance because it is intended to compensate for a loss of self but at the same time actually allows it to continue. True awareness of the reality of our prenatal experience on the other hand makes a more complete participation in life possible. The rupture in our life processes that occurs because of the traumatic aspect of birth and the lack of support in trying to overcome this must no longer be projected as alienation, as nothingness, as misery, or as earthly evil. It must no longer be suffered or fought against. Rather, seen as a human challenge and incentive for creative transformation, it can enrich our human existence. This is not only valid for the psychosocial sciences but also for the natural sciences, as the Austrian nuclear physicist Gerhard Grössing has shown (1994).

As a science, it seems to me that prenatal psychology can in a seminal way connect the unfortunate split between the humanities and natural science, which itself is a possible result of the traumatic aspects of birth and has split the unity of personal experience into purely mental and purely physical parts. Being prisoner in a body and feelings of nonphysicality are two sides of the same coin. René Descartes (1596–1650) stands at the outset of our modern thinking and feeling about life. He lost his mother when he was 1 year old and his father was not close to him. This may well have determined his view of the world, split between *res extensa* (the tangible mother to "touch") from which one is separated and the *res cognitans*, the self-awareness, the precociously developed *Ich*, the security of which compensates for the loss of the mother.

In a similar vein, the Jungian psychoanalyst Marie Luise von Franz (1952) writes: "Descartes did not trust life or himself or others at all. . . . It was definitely the early death of his mother which took away from him all optimism, all confidence in life and in his own feelings so that he encapsulated himself in the exclusive activity of his thinking" (p. 116). This personal fate and its resolution allowed him to name the projective, collective-psychological, existential predicament that had resulted from the loss of security in the Middle Ages and to propose spiritual alternatives. His personal experience of security in rationality blended itself with the contemporary communal quest for a new point of orientation. After a few dreams that were unquestionably birth dreams and deeply shook him, he gained a new, compensating security in his orientation on Ratio and Reason and with that he then formulated a new cultural paradigm. One of his biographers, Wolfgang Röd (1962), summarized the occurrence of his night of dreams and fever in late autumn 1619 as follows: "In an ecstatic experience, Descartes felt the spirit of truth descending upon him. This overpowered all threats from adversary forces to which he felt his philosophy was exposed" (p. 26). This describes the typical experience of rebirth that occurs after a spontaneous perinatal regression. It is also expressed in dreams in the course of which the dreamer, Descartes, is encircled by a storm as he walks through the streets and "is pressed irresistibly to one side by a whirlwind." Then follows a "shower of sparks" and "sounds like thunder" (p. 20).

The new worldview prepared by deep regression immortalized the split already mentioned between body and soul. The scientist also alienates himself from his own body in the same way. Edison's statement is the epitome of this: "I only need my body in order to carry my brain around" (quoted in Kutschmann 1986, p. 411). Such a statement makes it clear that we and our feelings toward life are at times exposed to the eccentric conditions of our birth and that our identity and attitude to life is liable to be malformed. An awareness of the powers and experience of the first phases of our life could help us to face this danger. In various psychotherapies, there is increasing hope that the clarification of our unconscious, of our birth trauma, primal pain, character armor— whatever we may call the primary malformation that occurs at the beginning of our life—can lead us to expanded awareness and a better founded humanity. However, this can only be successful when the hidden distortions in our so-called normal values become even more clear to us.

Fascism has shown us how disastrous a wanting-to-be-healthy and feeling healthy can be when it is in the service of a destructive ideal. Only a deeper understanding of the emergence and structuring of our cultural ideals can enable us to respond to the ecological tasks that lie before us. In recent years, we have experienced that positive developments here interlock and mutually strengthen each other. Improved economical conditions relieve the human relationship between the regressive reactivation of perinatal pain and the tendency to enact it in destructive social actions. This in turn sets energy free to improve our social and economical conditions. Thus, a positive feedback emerges that has contributed to the current favorable situation with social welfare systems and democratic rules in the Western Hemisphere.

However, it is my impression that the extent of psychological misery in our society is greatly underestimated. According to an epidemiological study carried out by Heinz Schepank (1987), a psychoanalyst from Mannheim, a third of the population suffers from an acute neurotic illness. About two million alcoholics live in Germany. The majority of the population live a life impaired by subacute neurotic and psychosomatic complaints. It is only since the 1960s that the human suffering expressed in alcoholism has actually been recognized as an illness. A general awareness that antisocial and criminal behavior is the result of deep suffering and stunted development from very earliest childhood onward has only come to light after the Second World War. Our attempt to manage suffering caused in our societies is limited to a legal, ritual-pragmatic, punitive response, because human social systems as a whole have so far not managed their problems adequately. Seen from a historical point of view, the times of naked hunger and the scourge of social catastrophe do not lie so far behind us.

It is my impression that our societies are still determined—far more than we are aware of—by the structures of military combat. This may be one of the reasons why the fundamental social task of providing supportive developmental opportunities for the next generation from its very beginning is only inadequately tackled. Young parents who face this task have at the same time the great burden of

228   The Fourth World of Mankind

establishing an existence in a competitive and achievement-oriented society. Disastrous negative feedback occurs in this situation. Because unborn and newborn babies are so stress sensitive, any pressure on the parents is immediately a handicap for their offspring from the beginning of the baby's life and limits its developmental chances. This again lays the foundations for restricted, obsessional, social systems. The next generation then faces the same initial conditions.

The findings of prenatal psychology question these inhibitive structures and prescribe a direction toward a transformation of our social ideals. In a peaceful society, the structures of combat should not play a significant role and, if at all, should serve the creation of dignified human life for the development of the next generation (Chamberlain 1993, Fedor-Freybergh 1983, Odent 1986). The reduction of the infant mortality rates and improved medical care during pregnancy are meritorious, but this only ensures bare survival.

Until now in our societies, the psychological dimension of life's beginning remains the concern of outsider movements. As the movement for gentle birth shows, the insights have only been put into action against the pressure of established structures. A change for the better can only occur when there is more general awareness of the significance of the experiences we all have gone through at the beginning of our life—an awareness that the heart of our experience, our soul, is fetal consciousness. Folk wisdom tells us, "That which comes from the sea, belongs to the sea." In modern terms, that which comes from the primal sea of the amniotic fluid must return. The same thing was symbolized in ancient Egypt in a sort of mythical, primal knowledge, in the representation of the soul as a bird with a human head and hands. Something of the floating that is an essential element of fetal experience is expressed here. It is this fetal consciousness as the root foundation of our soul to which we intuitively form a relationship and out of which we can, in creative moments, establish ourselves again and again.

Appendix:
The First Nine Months

ADVICE TO EXPECTANT PARENTS

From the many examples within this book, it is clear that the unborn child is already a human person with feelings, sensations, and perceptions. He or she is impressionable and inquisitive, and possesses the ability to learn, a desire to move, a natural identity, and emotional consciousness. Especially significant are in all probability the sense of balance, skin sensations, touch, taste, and hearing, as well as general coenaesthetic or holistic sensations and experiences. Besides the physiological-hormonal contact with the mother, a channel of intense, emotional communication also seems to exist through which living beings in close contact can instinctively perceive any mutual attraction or rejection. We have learned from premature babies about the elementary, emotional needs of unborn children. This sets the frame in which to give advice about how to treat a child before its birth, whereby a feeling for the needs of infants in the period immediately after birth can serve as a rough guide. What is important is to allow mother and child to decide the time to be born. Only about 5 percent of children are born on the calculated date of birth; 95 percent in the period of three weeks before to three weeks after this date (M. Klimek 1993, R. Klimek 1992, 1995).

Even in the prenatal phase of life, which appears to be so purely biological, a person is basically designed for self-realization through experience and in relationship. The reports of better condition after birth and of accelerated development in babies who received more care, of whatever sort, before birth are astonishing.

Emotional-relational nurture can be realized by the pre- and perinatal, haptonomic accompaniment, developed by Frans Veldman, who demonstrates that we all—and especially the child before birth—have the ability to establish a deep form of communication or affective contact. The mother can be shown how to make contact with her unborn child in this way and to invite it to move to a hand placed on the right side of the abdomen, and then to change to the left or also to move up or down. This can be easily perceived by changes in the silhouette of the abdomen, can be felt with the hands, or more objectively determined by ultrasound. The father can also make contact in this way. The parents can also develop a "swimming game" to which the child often spontaneously responds with knocking when it always occurs at a particular time and the child learns to expect it. This form of contact gains a special significance because it makes it possible for the mother to maintain contact with her child during the birth.

The currently most comprehensive concept of psychological antenatal care was presented by the American prenatal psychologist and psychotherapist Thomas Verny and the journalist Pamela Weintraub (1992) in their book *Nurturing the Unborn Child*. It contains exercises to encourage contact with the unborn child, making use of deep relaxation, visualization, directed use of the imagination, music, and stimulation by means of touch and speech. Of central importance are suggestions and exercises that deal with the development of parental identity and with the new, broader way in which individuals see themselves as a result of parenthood. The methods used include writing a diary, working on one's dreams, directed use of the imagination, dialogue with one's partner, making models, and so on. Another program from the United States is also designed to promote the relationship between the mother and her unborn child and was presented by the American psychologist Anne Jernberg (1988). The most important features of this program are as follows: "Draw a picture of yourself and the baby. Speak to and play with the baby. Tell the baby about the future when it will be grown up. Sing to the baby. . . . Tell the baby about its father. Tell the baby about the people it will meet when it has been born" (p. 257).

Voice, singing, and music play a special role in prenatal contact. The unborn child perceives everything very intensively and in great detail. After birth, the child shows special preferences and recognizes the voices of members of its family.

From this short summary, here is some advice for expectant parents:

1. Consider your child already before its birth to be a full-fledged member of your family with a special status.
2. Emotional nurture and intimacy promote the child's development and relationship abilities.
3. Nurture can take on the most diverse forms: stroking, speaking, listening to music, and general involvement in the life of the family.
4. Even before the birth, the father is an important person for the child.
5. General knowledge about prenatal development, which, for example, can be gained from picture books, can make the presence of the developing child emotionally more real.
6. The time invested in relating to the child during the pregnancy is rewarded by easier and unproblematic, postnatal development.
7. We live in a time in which the identities of men and women are changing. As a result, parents today must find their own, often completely new ways of dealing with the period of pregnancy relating to the unborn child and birth. A comprehensive literature is available to provide support (see References and APPPAH (the Association for Pre- and Perinatal Psychology and Health, 340 Colony Road, Box 994, Geyserville, CA 95441. Tel: 707–857–4041; Fax: 707–857–3764), and an increasing number of seminars make the rapid developments in our knowledge about the beginning of life more easily accessible.

References

To the reader: Where English translations of works cited in this reference list are available, they have been provided in parentheses following the German entries. Readers who are interested in accessing or clarifying German reference citations are invited to contact the author at Köpfelweg 52 / 69118 Heidelberg / Germany.

Adamson, L., and Tronick, E. (1980). *Babies as People: New Findings on Our Social Beginnings.* New York: Collier.

Adler, A. (1965). *Studien über die Minderwertigkeit von Organen.* Darmstadt: Wissenschaftliche Buchgemeinschaft.

Amendt, G., and Schwarz, M. (1992). *Das Leben unerwünschter Kinder.* Frankfurt/Main: Fischer.

Anand, K. J. S., and Hickey, P. R. (1987). Pain and its effects in the human neonate and fetus. *The New England Journal of Medicine* 317:1321–1329.

Arnold, D. (1996). "If we weren't for these pictures . . ."—Joseph Beuys. *International Journal of Prenatal and Perinatal Psychology and Medicine* 8:47–56.

APPPAH (Association for Pre- and Perinatal Psychology and Health). (1996). *One Hundred Books (and Videos) in Pre- and Perinatal Psychology and Health: 1975–1995.* Geyserville, CA: APPPAH.

Bächtold-Stäubli, H., ed. (1987a). *Handwörterbuch des deutschen Aberglaubens,* vol. 6. Berlin: deGruyter.

—— 1987b). *Handwörterbuch des deutschen Aberglaubens,* vol. 7. Berlin: deGruyter.

—— (1987c). *Handwörterbuch des deutschen Aberglaubens,* vol. 8. Berlin: deGruyter.

Bair, D. (1991). *Samuel Beckett: Eine Biographie.* Hamburg: Rowohlt. ([1978] *Samuel Beckett: A Biography.* London: Jonathan Cape.)

Beckett, S. (1976a). *Warten auf Godot.* (*Waiting for Godot*) In *Werke* I. 1. Frankfurt/Main: Suhrkamp.

—— (1976b). *Alle, die da fallen.* (*All that Falls*) In *Werke* I. 2. Frankfurt/Main: Suhrkamp.

Benedetti, G. (1983a). Praenatale Psychologie und Persönlichkeit im Lichte der analytischen Untersuchung von erwachsenen Kindern psychotischer Mütter. Festvortrag zum 60. Geburtstag von Theodor Hau. (unpublished lecture).

—— (1983b). *Todeslandschaften der Seele.* Göttingen: Vandenhoeck and Ruprecht.

Bennholdt-Thomsen, A., and Guzzoni, A. (1990). Zur Theorie des Verstehens im 18 Jahrhundert. In *Klio und Psyche,* ed. T. Kornbichler. Pfaffenweiler: Centaurus.

Bergh, B. van den. (1990). The influence of maternal emotions during pregnancy on fetal and neonatal behavior. *Pre- and Perinatal Psychology* 5:119–130.

Bettelheim, B. (1977). *Kinder brauchen Märchen.* Stuttgart: Deutsche Verlags-Anstalt. (*The Uses of Enchantment.* New York: Knopf, 1976.)

Bick, C. (1986). *Neurohypnose.* Frankfurt/Main: Ullstein.

Bieback, K. (1991). Glück and Unglück im Geburts—und Vorge-burtserleben. In *Erscheinungsweisen pränatalen und perinatalen Erlebens in den psychotherapeutischen Settings*, ed. L. Janus. Heidelberg: Textstudio Gross.

Blarer, S. (1982). Manifestation einer Geburtskomplikation in Träumen und Phantasien. In *Geburt—Eintritt in eine neue Welt*, ed. S. Schindler. Göttingen: Verlag für Psychologie.

Blazy, H. (1991a). Ich lasse meinen Geist wandern. Schwangerschaft und Geburt in Darstellungen der modernen indonesischen Literatur. In *Die kulturelle Verarbeitung pränatalen und perinatalen Erlebens*, ed. L. Janus. Heidelberg: Textstudio Gross.

——— (1991b). On premature delivery, seen through the mirror of transference and countertransference in child psychotherapy. *International Journal of Prenatal and Perinatal Studies* 3:119–124.

Blum, T., ed. (1993). *Prenatal Perception, Learning and Bonding*. Heidelberg: Textstudio Gross.

Bolle, R. (1991). Zur kulturellen Integration von prä- und perinatalen Erlebnisfeldern am Beispiel vom Umgang mit psychoaktiven Substanzen. In *Die kulturelle Verarbeitung pränatalen und perinatalen Erlebens*, ed. L. Janus. Heidelberg: Textstudio Gross.

Brinton, D. (1894). Nagualism. In *Proceedings of the American Philosophical Society* 33:11–73.

Brosch, R., and Rust, M. (1989). Schmerz und Anaesthesie bei Früh- und Neugeborenen. *Anaesthesiologie und Intensivmedizin* 10:287–291, 11:334–338.

Bürgin, D. (1982). Uber einige Aspekte der pränatalen Entwicklung. In *Psychiatrie des Säuglings—und Kleinkindalters*, ed. G. Nissen. Bern: Huber.

Burkert, W. (1990). *Wilder Ursprung. Opferritual und Mythos bei den Griechen*. Berlin: Wagenbach.

Campe, J. H. (1985). *Uber die früheste Bildung junger Kinderseelen*. Frankfurt/Main: Ullstein.

Cardinal, M. (1977). *Les mots pour le dire*. New York: French and European Publications.

Carus, C. G. (1846). *Psyche—Zur Entwicklungsgeschichte der Seele.* Pforzheim: Flammer und Hoffmann.

Chamberlain, D. (1983). *Consciousness at Birth: A Review of the Empirical Evidence.* San Diego, CA: Chamberlain Communications.

——— (1990). *Woran Babys sich erinnern.* Munich: Kosel. (*Babies Remember Birth.* New York: St. Martin's, 1988.)

——— (1993). How pre- and perinatal psychology can transform the world. *International Journal of Prenatal and Perinatal Studies* 5:413–424.

Cheek, D. (1974). Sequential head and shoulder movements appearing with age-regression in hypnosis to birth. *American Journal of Clinical Hypnosis* 16:261–266.

Clauser, G. (1971). *Die vorgeburtliche Entstehung der Sprache.* Stuttgart: Enke.

Compayré, J. G. (1900). *Die Entwicklung der Kinderseele.* (*The Development of the Child's Psyche*) Altenburg: Oskar Bonde.

Condon, W., and Sander, L. (1974). Synchrony demonstrated between movements of the neonate and adult speech. *Child Development* 45:456–462.

Conrad, K. (1966). *Die beginnende Schizophrenie.* Stuttgart: Thieme.

Costa Segui, M. (1995). The prenatal period as the origin of character structures. *International Journal of Prenatal and Perinatal Psychology and Medicine* 7:309–322.

Cranston Anderson, G., et al. (1986). Kangaroo care for premature infants. *American Journal of Nursing* 86:807–809.

Cremerius, J., ed. (1988). *Untergangsphantasien.* Würzburg: Königshausen und Neumann.

Crisan, H. (1994). The perinatal psychosomatic aspects of Kundalini-Yoga. *International Journal of Prenatal and Perinatal Psychology and Medicine* 6:547–579.

Cullen, J. H., and Connolly, J. (1987). The effects of some physical and psychosocial prenatal stressors on early development. In *Perspectives on Stress and Stress-Related Topics.* Heidelberg: Springer.

Dalí, S. (1973). *So wird man Dalí.* Rastatt: Moewig.

————— (1984). *Das geheime Leben des Salvador Dalí.* Munich: Schirmer/Mosel.

Davidson, J. (1985). The shadow of life: psychosocial explanations for placenta rituals. *Culture, Medicine and Psychiatry* 9:75–92.

Davies, N. (1981). *Human Sacrifice.* New York: William Morrow.

DeCasper, A., and Fifer, W. (1980). Of human bonding: newborns prefer their mothers' voices. *Science* 208:1174–1176.

DeMause, L. (1979a). *Hört ihr die Kinder weinen.* Frankfurt/Main: Suhrkamp. (*The History of Childhood.* New York: The Psychohistory Press, 1974.)

————— (1979b). Psychohistory. In *Kindheit* 1:59ff.

————— (1989a). *Psychohistorie.* Frankfurt/Main: Suhrkamp. (*Foundations of Psychohistory.* New York: Creative Roots, 1982.)

————— (1989b). Fötale Ursprünge der Geschichte. ("Fetal Origins of History") In *Psychohistorie.* Frankfurt/Main: Suhrkamp.

————— (1991). The Gulf War as a mental disorder. *The Journal of Psychohistory* 19:1–22.

————— (1996). The origins of war and social violence. *The Journal of Psychohistory* 23:344–391.

deSnoo, K. (1942). *Das Problem der Menschwerdung im Lichte der vergleichenden Geburtshilfe.* Jena: Gustav Fischer.

Diallina, M. (1987). Psychotherapeutische Wiedergeburt im psychotischen Dasein. In *Pränatale und Perinatale Psychologie und Medizin,* ed. P. Fedor-Freybergh. Berlin: Rotation Verlag.

Dörner, G. (1987). Bedeutung der hormonabhängigen Gehirnentwicklung und der prä- und frühpostnatalen Psychophysiologie für die Präventivmedizin. In *Pränatale und Perinatale Psychologie und Medizin,* ed. P. Fedor-Freybergh. Berlin: Rotation Verlag. (Significance of hormone-dependent brain development and pre- and early postnatal psychophysiology for preventive medicine. In *Prenatal and Perinatal Psychology and Medicine,* ed. P. Fedor-Freybergh and V. Vogel. Casterton Hall: Parthenon.

————— (1988). Bedeutung der hormonabhängigen Gehirnentwicklung für die Ontogenese. In *Das Leben vor und während der Geburt*, ed. G. Schusser and W. Hartzmann. Osnabrück: Universitätsdruck Osnabrück.

Dowling, T. (1987a). Die Bedeutung prä- und perinataler Erfahrungen in der Kindertherapie. *Kind und Umwelt* 56:20–35.

———— (1987b). Personal communication.

———— (1988). The psychological significance of the placenta. In *Das Leben vor und während der Geburt*, ed. G. Schusser and W. Hatzmann. Osnabrück: Universitätsdruck Osnabrück.

———— (1990). The roots of the collective unconscious. In *Das Seelenleben der Ungeborenen—eine Wurzel unseres Unbewußten*. Pfaffenweiler: Centaurus.

———— (1991a). Pränatale Regression in der Hypnose. In *Erscheinungsweisen pränatalen und perinatalen Erlebens in den psychotherapeutischen Settings*, ed. L. Janus. Heidelberg: Textstudio Gross.

———— (1991b). Pränatale und perinatale Aspekte des Zweiten Weltkrieges. In *Die kulturelle Verarbeitung pränatalen und perinatalen Erlebens*, ed. L. Janus. Heidelberg: Textstudio Gross.

———— (1992). Models of birth in psychotherapy. In *Pre- and Peri-Natal Psycho-Medicine*, ed. R. Klimek. Cracow: DWN DReAM.

———— (1994). Wir lieben nur, wovon wir träumen. In *Ungewollte Kinder*, ed. H. Häsing and L. Janus. Reinbek: Rowohlt.

Dudenhausen, J., and Saling, E., eds. (1990). *Perinatale Medizin*. Stuttgart: Thieme.

Egli, H. (1982). *Das Schlangensymbol*. Olten: Walter.

Eichenberger, E. (1987). Hinweise auf prä- und perinatale Störungen im anamnestischen Gespräch. In *Pränatale und Perinatale Psychologie und Medizin*, ed. P. Fedor-Freybergh. Berlin: Rotation Verlag.

Eissler, K. R. (1978). Creativity and adolescence. *Psychoanalytic Study of the Child* 33:461–517. New Haven, CT: Yale University Press.

Eliade, M. (1960). Mythos und Symbol des Seiles. In *Eranos Jahrbuch* 29. Zurich: Rhein Verlag.

———— (1966). *Rites and Symbols of Initiation: The Mysteries of Birth and Rebirth.* New York: HarperCollins.

———— (1968). *Kosmos und Geschichte.* Frankfurt/Main: Suhrkamp.

———— (1985). *Yoga.* Frankfurt/Main: Suhrkamp. ([1989] *Yoga: Immortality and Freedom.* New York: Viking Penguin.)

———— (1986). *Die Religionen und das Heilige.* Frankfurt/Main: Suhrkamp.

———— (1988). *Das Mysterium der Wiedergeburt.* Frankfurt/Main: Suhrkamp.

Emerson, W. (1989). Psychotherapy with infants and children. *Pre- and Perinatal Psychology Journal* 3:190–217.

———— (1996). The vulnerable prenate. *Pre- and Perinatal Psychology Journal* 10:125–142.

Eschenbach, U. (1994). Die Spiegelung frühen Leids im Bild. In *Ungewolte Kinder,* ed. H. Häsing and L. Janus. Reinbek: Rowohlt.

Fabricius, J. (1989). *Alchemy.* Wellingborough: The Aquarian Press.

———— (1991). Pränatale und perinatale Motive in der Malerei. In *Die kulturelle Verarbeitung präntalen und perinatalen Erlebens,* ed. L. Janus. Heidelberg: Textstudio Gross.

Fedor-Freybergh, P. (1983). Psychophysische Gegebenheiten der Perinatalzeit als Umwelt des Kindes. In *Ökologie der Perinatalzeit,* ed. S. Schindler and H. Zimprich. Stuttgart: Hippokrates.

————, ed. (1987). *Pränatale und Perinatale Psychologie und Medizin.* Berlin: Rotation Verlag.

———— (1989). The International Society of Prenatal and Perinatal Psychology and Medicine. *International Journal of Prenatal and Perinatal Studies* 2:139–144.

Fedor-Freybergh, P., and Vogel, V., eds. (1988). *Prenatal and Perinatal Psychology and Medicine.* Casterton Hall: Parthenon.

Ferenczi, S. (1964a). Entwicklungsstufen des Wirklichkeitssinnes. In *Bausteine der Psychoanalyse,* vol. 1. Bern: Huber.

———— (1964b). Uber den Anfall der Epileptiker. In *Bausteine der Psychoanalyse,* vol. 3. Bern: Huber.

Ferreira, A. (1960). The pregnant woman's emotional attitude and its reflection on the newborn. *American Journal of Orthopsychiatry* 30:553–561.

Field, T. (1982). Discrimination and imitation of facial expressions by neonates. *Science* 218:179–181.

Findeisen, B. (1992). The long-term psychological impact of pre- and perinatal experiences. In *Prenatal and Perinatal Psycho-Medicine*, ed. R. Klimek. Cracow: DWN DReAM.

Fischle, W. (1982). *Der Weg sur Mitte.* Stuttgart: Belser.

Fitzpatrick, M. P. (1988). Pre- and perinatal stress: the psychotic individual. *Pre- and Perinatal Psychology Journal* 2:258–269.

Fodor, N. (1949). *The Search for the Beloved: A Clinical Investigation of the Trauma of Birth and Prenatal Conditions.* New York: University Books.

Foresti, G. (1982). Mütterliche Angst und Zustände kindlicher Ubererregbarkeit. In *Pränatale und Perinatale Psychosomatik*, ed. T. Hau and S. Schindler. Stuttgart: Hippokrates.

Föster, M., ed. (1984). *Jürgen Bartsch—Nachruf auf eine Bestie.* Essen: Torso.

Frankfort, H. (1942). *Kinship and the Gods.* Chicago: University of Chicago Press.

Franz, von, M-L. (1952). *Der Traum des Descartes*, Zurich: Rascher.

Freud, S. (1963). Hemmung, Symptom and Angst. *Gesammelte Werke*, vol. 14. Frankfurt/Main: Fischer. (Inhibitions, symptoms, and anxiety. *Standard Edition* 20.)

———— (1966a). Analyse der Phobie eines funfjährigen Knaben. *Gesammelte Werke*, vol. 7. Frankfurt/Main: Fischer. (Analysis of a phobia of a five-year-old boy. *Standard Edition* 10.)

———— (1966b). Vorlesungen zur Einführung in die Psychoanalyse. *Gesammelte Werke*, vol. 11. Frankfurt/Main: Fischer. (Introductory lectures on psycho-analysis. *Standard Edition* 16.)

———— (1966c). Aus der Geschichte einer infantilen Neurose. *Gesammelte Werke*, vol. 12. Frankfurt/Main: Fischer. (From the history of an infantile neurosis. *Standard Edition* 17.)

———— (1972). Die Traumdeutung. *Studienausgabe*, vol. 2.

Frankfurt/Main: Fischer. (The interpretation of dreams. *Standard Edition* 4/5.)

Freud, W. E. (1988). The concept of cathexis and its usefulness for prenatal psychology. In *Prenatal and Perinatal Psychology and Medicine*, ed. F. Fedor-Freybergh and V. Vogel. Casterton Hall: Parthenon.

Friedrich, B. (1993). Pra- und Perinatales Erleben—Inszenierungen in Kindertherapien. *International Journal of Prenatal and Perinatal Psychology and Medicine* 5:383–388.

——— (1996). "Riß in der Beziehung"—Gedanken uber die Therapie eines Sechsjährigen der zu früh geboren wurde. *International Journal of Prenatal and Perinatal Psychology and Medicine* 8:65–72.

Galati, A. (1996). "A Time to Be Reborn"—a case report. *International Journal of Prenatal and Perinatal Psychology and Medicine* 8:21–26.

Gareis, B., and Wiesnet, E. (1974). *Frühkindheit und Kriminalität.* Munich: Goldmann.

Garley, D. (1924). Uber den Schock des Geborenwerdens. ("The Shock of Being Born") *Internationale Zeitschrift für Psychoanalyse*, vol. 10:135–163.

Gehrts, H. (1966a). Drachenzug und Bruderkampf: Untersuchungen zur Polspannung im Königsritual. *Antaios* 7:166–195.

——— (1966b). Schamanistische Elemente im Zaubermärchen. In *Schamanentum und Zaubermärchen*, ed. H. Gehrts and G. Lademann-Priemer. Kassel: Erich Röth.

——— (1967). *Das Märchen und das Opfer.* Bonn: Bouvier.

Gehrts, H., and Lademann-Priemer, G., eds. (1966). *Schamanentum und Zaubermärchen.* Kassel: Erich Röth.

Gélis, J. (1989). *Die Geburt.* Munich: Diederichs.

Genazzini, A. (1989). Ontogeny of fetal opioids and their secretion at birth. Ref. 9. International Congress of JSPPM in Jerusalem.

Goethe, J. W., von. (1967a). West-östlicher Divan. In *Goethes Werke*, vol. 2. Hamburg: Wegener.

——— (1967b). Faust. In *Goethes Werke*, vol. 3. Hamburg: Wegener.

——— (1967c). Dichtung und Wahrheit. In *Goethes Werke*, vol. 9. Hamburg: Wegener.

Graber, G. H. (1924). *Die Ambivalent des Kindes*. Leipzig: Internationaler Psychoanalytischer Verlag.

——— (1966). *Die Not des Lebens und ihre Überwindung*. Düsseldorf: Ardschuna.

———, ed. (1974). *Pränatale Psychologie*. Munich: Kindler.

——— (1978a). Ursprung, Zwiespalt und Einheit der Seele. In *Gesammelte Schriften*, vol. 1. Berlin: Pinel.

——— (1978b). Das Unbewußte bei Carus. In *Gesammelte Schriften*, vol. 3. Berlin: Pinel.

——— (1978c). Zur Lehre der Psychotherapie. In *Gesammelte Schriften*, vol. 3. Berlin: Pinel.

Grant, M. (1982). *Die Gladiatoren*. Frankfurt/Main: Ullstein.

Greenacre, P. (1945). The biological economy of birth. *Psychoanalytic Study of the Child* 1:31–51. New York: International Universities Press.

Grimm, J., and Grimm, W. (1969). *Kinder- und Hausmärchen*. Munich: Winkler. (*The Classic Grimm's Fairy Tales*. Philadelphia: Courage Books, 1989.)

Grinspoon, L., and Bakalar, J. B., eds. (1983). *Psychedelic Reflections*. New York: Human Sciences.

Grof, S. (1983). Perinatale Ursprünge von Kriegen, Revolutionen und Totalitarismus. *Kindheit* 5:25–40.

——— (1985). *Geburt, Transzendenz, Tod*. Munich: Kösel.

——— (1988). *Topographie des Unbewußten: LSD im Dienst der tiefenpsychologischen Forschung*. Stuttgart: Klett-Cotta. (*Realms of the Human Unconscious*. New York: Viking, 1975.)

Gross, W. (1982). *Was erkebt das Kind im Mutterleib?* Freiburg: Herder.

Grössing, G. (1994). The uterus sky as model and preexisting image in natural science. *International Journal of Prenatal and Perinatal Psychology and Medicine* 6:315–335.

Grözinger, W. (1984). *Kinder kritzeln, zeichnen, malen*. Munich: Prestel.

Gsell, E. (1995). Es ist Zeit, geborn zu werden. *International Journal of Prenatal and Perinatal Psychology and Medicine* 7:337–366.

Gupta, D., and Gupta, D. (1989). Fertilisation and prenatal development of body and mind: ancient Indian medical observations. *International Journal of Prenatal and Perinatal Studies* 1:7–19.

Hakanson, T. (1988). Cross-cultural descriptions of prenatal experience. In *Prenatal and Perinatal Psychology and Medicine*, ed. P. Fedor-Freybergh and V. Vogel. Casterton Hall: Parthenon.

Harner, M. (1982). *Der Weg des Schamanen*. Reinbek: Rowohlt. (*Way of the Shaman*. New York: Bantam, 1982.)

Häsing, H., and Janus, L. (1994). *Ungewolte Kinder*. Reinbek: Rowohlt.

Hau, E. (1974). Prä- und perinatale Milieufaktoren als Ursachen für die Beunruhigung der Nachkriegsgeneration. In *Pränatale Psychologie*, ed., G. H. Graber. Munich: Kindler.

Hau, T. (1982). Narzißmus und Intentionalitat prä- und perinataler Aspekte. In *Pränatale und Perinatale Psychosomatik*, ed. T. Hau and S. Schindler. Stuttgart: Hippokrates.

Heidegger, M. (1986). *Sein und Zeit*. Tübingen: Max Niemeyer. (*Being and Time*. San Francisco: Harper, 1962.)

Heimann, P. (1989). Notes on early development. In *About Children and Children-No-Longer*. London: Routledge.

Hellon, C. (1980). Suicide and age in Alberta, Canada, 1951–1977. *Archives of General Psychology* 37:502–523.

Hepper, P. G. (1995). Human fetal "olfactory" learning. *International Journal of Prenatal and Perinatal Psychology and Medicine* 7:147–151.

Hermsen, E. (1993). Regression ad uterum: the embryological symbolism of the ancient Egyptian beyond and pre- and perinatal psychology. *International Journal of Prenatal and Perinatal Psychology and Medicine* 5:361–382.

——— (1996). Death as birth: the ancient Egyptian beyond, the unconscious, and the lake of flame. *International Journal of Prenatal and Perinatal Psychology and Medicine* 8:243–258.

Hoffmann, E. T. A. (1967). *Das Fräulein von Scuderi.* (*The Woman from Scuderi.*) Werke Bd. 2. Frankfurt/Main: Insel.

Hoffmann, J. (1988). Popmusik, Pubertät, Narißmus. *Psyche* 42:961–980.

Hollos, I. (1924). Die Psychoneurose eines Frühgeborenen. *Internationale Zeitschrift für ärztliche Psychoanalyse* 10:423–433.

Hollweg, W. H. (1990). Psychosomatische Symptome in der Muskulatur und im Skelett. In *Das Seelenleben der Ungeborenen—eine Wurzel unseres Unbewußten.* Pfaffenweiler: Centaurus.

——— (1995). Von der Wahrheit, die frei macht. Heidelberg: Mattes.

Homer. (1979). *Ilias.* Munich: dtv. (*The Iliad.* New York: Doubleday, 1989).

Hornung, E. (1968). *Altägyptische Höllenvorstellungen.* Berlin: Akademie-Verlag.

——— (1971). *Der Eine und die Vielen.* Darmstadt: Wissenschaftliche Buchgemeinschaft.

——— (1984). *Ägyptische Unterweltsbücher.* Zurich: Artemis.

——— (1985). *Tal der Könige.* Zurich: Artemis.

Horowitz, M. J. (1976). *Stress Response Syndromes.* New York: Jason Aronson.

Huber, R. (1994). Die wiedergefundene vorgeburtliche Beziehung. *International Journal of Prenatal and Perinatal Psychology and Medicine* 6:141–150.

——— (1995). Die prä- und perinatale Dimension erweitert die Möglichkeiten unseres analytischen Verstehens. *International Journal of Prenatal and Perinatal Psychology and Medicine* 7:499–508.

Hubert, H., and Mauss, M. (1968). *Sacrifice—Its Nature and Function.* London: Cohen and West.

Hungar, B. (1996). Brutkastenerfahrung—Verletzung des Selbst: Klaus M. *International Journal of Prenatal and Perinatal Psychology and Medicine* 8:85–88.

Ianniruberto, A., and Tajani, E. (1981). Ultrasonic study of fetal movements. *Seminars in Perinatology* 5:175–181.

Ingalls, P. M. S. (1996). Birth memories, psychotherapy, and philosophy. *International Journal of Prenatal and Perinatal Psychology and Medicine* 8:157–170.

Irving, M. (1989). Natalism as pre- and perinatal metaphor. *Pre- and Perinatal Psychology* 4:83–110.

Jacobson, B. (1988). Perinatal origin of eventual self-destructive behavior. *Pre- and Perinatal Psychology* 2:227–241.

Janov, A. (1974). *Das befreite Kind.* Frankfurt/Main: Fischer. (*The Feeling Child.* New York: Simon & Schuster, 1973.)

——— (1984). *Frühe Prägungen.* Frankfurt/Main: Fischer. (*Imprints: The Lifelong Effects of the Birth Experience.* New York: Coward McCann, 1983.)

Janus, L. (1987). Psychoanalysis and stress. In *Perspectives on Stress and Stress-Related Topics*, ed. F. Lolas and H. Mayer. Heidelberg: Springer.

——— (1988). The trauma of birth as reflected in the psychoanalytic process. In *Prenatal and Perinatal Psychology and Medicine*, ed. P. Fedor-Freybergh and V. Vogel. Casterton Hall: Parthenon.

——— (1989a). Perinatale Wurzeln psychosomatischer Symptombildungen. In *Soziopsychosomatik*, ed. W. Söllner. Heidelberg: Springer.

——— (1989b). The hidden dimension of prenatal and perinatal experience in the works of Freud, Jung and Klein. *International Journal of Prenatal and Perinatal Studies* 1:51–65.

——— (1990a). Haptonomische Aspekte in Kleists Marionettentheater. In *Öffnung zum Leben.* Festschrift, Frans Veldman, dem Begründer der Haptonomie, gewidmet, ed. M. Knaapen, et al. Overasselt: Stichting.

——— (1990b). *Die Psychoanalyse der vorgeburtlichen Lebenszeit und der Geburt.* Pfaffenweiler: Centaurus.

———, ed. (1990c). *Das Seelenleben des Ungeborenen—eine Wurzel unseres Unbewußten.* Pfaffenweiler: Centaurus.

——— (1990d). Fantasies of regression to the womb and rebirth as the central elements of the psychotherapeutic process.

International Journal of Prenatal and Perinatal Studies 2:89–100.

———, ed. (1991a). *Erscheinungsweisen pränatalen und perinatalen Erlebens in den psychotherapeutischen Settings.* Heidelberg: Textstudio Gross.

——— (1991b). Die frühe Ich-Entwicklung im Spiegel der LSD-Psychotherapie von Athanassios Kafkalides. *Zeitschrift für Individualpsychologie* 16:111–124.

———, ed. (1991c). *Die kulturelle Verarbeitung pränatalen und perinatalen Erlebens.* Heidelberg: Textstudio Gross.

——— (1991d). Psychologische Aspekte der Frühgeburt. *Kind und Umwelt* 70:10–22.

——— (1991e). Prä- und perinatale Aspekte in Freuds Krankengeschichten des Kindes—und Jugendalters. In *Aller Anfang ist schwer,* ed. C. Büttner, Elschenbroich, and A. Ende. Weinheim: Beltz.

——— (1993a). The relationship of pre- and perinatal psychology to 20th century art, literature, and philosophy. *Pre- and Perinatal Psychology Journal* 8:129–147.

——— (1993b). Prenatal psychology and perinatal medicine. In *2nd World Congress of Perinatal Medicine Proceedings,* ed. E. V. Cosmi and G. C. DiRenzo. Bologna: Monduzzi Editore.

——— (1994). Das verleugnete Leid der deutschen Kriegskinder. In *Ungewollte Kinder,* ed. H. Häsing and L. Janus. Reinbek: Rowohlt.

——— (1995a). Prenatal psychology, culture and war. *The Journal of Psychohistory* 22:461–480.

——— (1995b). The prenatal dimension: its relevance to psychosomatic obstetrics. In *Psychosomatic Obstetrics and Gynaecology,* ed. J. Bitzer and M. Stauber. Bologna: Editore Monduzzi.

Janus, L., and Maiwald, M. (1992). Entwicklung, Verhalten und Erleben in der Pränatalzeit und die Folgen für die Lebensgeschichte–Eine bibliographische Übersicht. *International Journal of Prenatal and Perinatal Studies* 4:101–140.

Jernberg, A. (1988). Promoting prenatal and perinatal mother–

child bonding. In *Prenatal and Perinatal Psychology and Medicine*. Casterton Hall: Parthenon.

Jones, E. (1923). Anxiety and birth. *International Journal of Psycho-Analysis* 4:120.

Jones, E. (1985). Anorexia nervosa, bulimia and birth. *Psychology Bulletin* 6:1–6.

Kafkalides, A. (1995). *The Knowledge of the Womb*. Heidelberg: Mattes.

Kakar, S. (1984). *Schamanen, Heilige und Arzte*. Munich: Biederstein.

Kantorowicz, E. (1990). *Die zwei Körper des Königs*. Munich: dtv. (*The King's Two Bodies*. Princeton, NJ: Princeton University Press, 1957.)

Keppler, K., et al. (1979). Die frühkindliche Anamnese der Schizophrenen. *Nervenarzt* 50:719–724.

Kilbridge, J. (1990). Sociocultural factors and perinatal development of Baganda infants: the precocity issue. *Pre- and Perinatal Psychology* 4:281–300.

Klaus, M. H., and Kennel, J. H. (1983). *Mutter-Kind-Bindung. Über die Folgen einer frühen Trennung*. Munich: Kösel. (*Maternal–Infant Bonding*. St. Louis, MO: C. V. Mosby, 1976.)

Klee, P. (1975). *Die Ordnung der Dinge*. Stuttgart: Hatje.

Klimek, M. (1993). Psychological aspects of determining the expected date of delivery. *International Journal of Prenatal and Perinatal Psychology and Medicine* 5:143–150.

Klimek, R. (1992). *Prenatal and Perinatal Medicine*. Cracow: DWN DReAM.

Klimek, R., Fedor-Freybergh, P., Janus, L., and Walas-Skolicka, E., eds. (1996). *A Time to Be Born*. Heidelberg: Mattes.

Klimek, R., and Walas-Skolicka, E. (1995). Birth term in terms of psycho-medicine. *International Journal of Prenatal and Perinatal Psychology and Medicine* 7:3–6.

Kluge, F. (1967). *Etymologisches Wörterbuch der deutschen Sprache*. Berlin: deGruyter.

Knaapen, M., et al., eds. (1990). *Öffnung zum Leben*. Festschrift,

Frans Veldman, dem Begründer der Haptonomie, gewidmet. Overasselt: Stichting.

Köhler, A. (1986). *Wiedergeburt und Kreissymbol—Ein Erfahrungsbericht aus den Erfahrungsbereichen des Zen und des intuitiven Atmens.* Kirchzarten: Author's edition.

Kohut, H., ed. (1977). *Introspektion, Empathie und Psychoanalyse.* Frankfurt/Main: Suhrkamp.

Kohut, H., and Levarie, S. (1977). Über den Musikgenuß. In *Introspektion, Empathie und Psychoanalyse*, ed. H. Kohut. Frankfurt/Main: Suhrkamp.

Kolata, G. (1984). Studying learning in the womb. *Science* 225:302ff.

Kornbichler, T., ed. (1990). *Klio und Psyche.* Pfaffenweiler: Centaurus.

Kraft, H. (1988). "Der Demiurg ist ein Zwitter"—Aspekte der Initiation im Roman. In *Untergansphantasien*, ed. J. Cremerius. Würzburg: Königshausen und Neumann.

——— (1991). Die Rituale der Initiation in den Performances von Joseph Beuys und Peter Gilles. In *Die kulturelle Verarbeitung pränatalen und perinatalen Erlebens*, ed. L. Janus. Heidelberg: Textstudio Gross.

Kruse, F. (1969). *Die Anfänge des menschlichen Seelenlebens.* Stuttgart: Enke.

Kubin, A. (1909). *Die andere Seite.* Munich: Edition Spangenburg.

Kugele, D. (1990). Perinatale Zusammenhänge bei Enkopresis. In *Das Seelenleben des Ungeborenen—eine Wurzel unseres Unbewußten*, ed. L. Janus. Heidelberg: Textstudio Gross.

Kuntner, L. (1986). Die Geburtshilfe in der europäischen Volksmedizin. *Hessische Blätter fur Volks- und Kulturforschung* 19:123–138.

Kupperberg, P. (1980). *Die Vernichtung Kryptons.* Stuttgart: Ehapa.

Kurrek, H. (1986). Das Geburtstrauma. Aspekte im Wandel der Medizin. *Acta Medica Empirica* 35:304–310.

——— (1987). Das Geburtstrauma—Evolutionsbedingte Pathologie. *Acta Empirica* 36:278–280.

——— (1988). Ist das Geburtstrauma unvermeidlich? *Raum und Zeit* 36:32–34.

Kussmann, T. (1977). Pawlow und das klassische Konditionieren. In *Pawlow und die Folgen*, ed. H. Zeier. Zürich: Kindler.

Kutschmann, W. (1986). *Der Naturwissenschaftler und sein Körper.* Frankfurt/Main: Suhrkamp.

Lake, F. (1979). *Studies in Constricted Confusion.* Unpublished manuscript.

Landsman, S. G. (1989). Metaphors: the language of pre- and perinatal trauma. *Pre- and Perinatal Psychology* 4:33–42.

Leboyer, F. (1986). *Geburt ohne Gewalt.* Munich: Kösel.

Lempp, R., ed. (1984). *Psychische Entwicklung und Schizophrenie.* Bern: Huber.

Lester, B., and Boukydis, C., eds. (1985). *Infant Crying.* New York: Plenum.

Leyh, C. (1996). Die Wiederbelebung prä- und perinataler Traumatisierungen in der analytischen Arbeit mit Kindern und Jugenlichen. *International Journal of Prenatal and Perinatal Psychology and Medicine* 8:73–84.

Liley, M., and Day, B. (1967). *Moderne Mutterschaft.* Berne: Phoenix/Scherz.

Lind, J., and Truby, H. (1965). Cry sounds of the newborn infant. In *Newborn Infant Cry*, ed. J. Lind. *Acta Paediatrica Scandinavica*, 163, Suppl.

Lolas, F., and Mayer, H., eds. (1987). *Perspectives on Stress and Stress-Related Topics.* Heidelberg: Springer.

Long, C. (1963). The placenta in lore and legend. *Bulletin of the Medical Library Association* 51:233–241.

Lou, H. C. (1989). Endogenous opioids may protect the perinatal brain hypoxia. *Developmental Pharmacology and Therapy* 13:129–133.

Ludwig, B. (1983). Postmortem CT and autopsy in perinatal intracranial hemorrhage. *AJNR* 4:27–36.

Lukesch, H. (1981). *Schwangerschafts- und Geburtsängste.* Stuttgart: Enke.

Macfarlane, A. (1978). *Die Geburt.* Stuttgart: Klett-Cotta. (*The Psychology of Childbirth.* Cambridge, MA: Harvard University Press, 1977.)

Macho, T. (1989). Heideggers Todesbegriff. *Manuskripte* 104:37–47.

Mahler, M., et al. (1978). *Die psychische Geburt des Menschen.* Frankfurt/Main: Fischer.

Maiwald, M. (1994). Development, behavior, and psychic experience in the prenatal period and the consequences for life history. *International Journal of Prenatal Psychology and Medicine* 6/Suppl.: 1–48.

Maiwald, M., and Janus, L. (1993). Development, behavior, and psychic experience in the prenatal period and the consequences for life history—a bibliographic survey. *International Journal of Prenatal and Perinatal Psychology and Medicine* 5:451–485.

Malebranche, N. (1674). *Erforschung der Wahrheit,* vol. 1. Munich: Buchenau, 1914.

Marnie, E. (1989). *Pre-Birth Bonding.* Carson, CA: Hay House.

Masson, J. (1986). *Sigmund Freud Briefe an Wilhelm Fließ.* Frankfurt/Main: Fischer.

Matejcek, Z. (1987). Kinder aus unerwünschter Schwangerschaft geboren: Longitudinale Studie über 20 Jahre. In *Pränatale und Perinatale Psychologie und Medizin,* ed. P. Fedor-Freybergh. Berlin: Rotation Verlag.

Mauger, B. (1995). Birth as metaphor: childbirth as initiation and transformation. *International Journal of Prenatal and Perinatal Psychology and Medicine* 7:465–474.

Maur, K., ed. (1989). *Salvador Dalí.* Stuttgart: Hatje.

Meifert, A., and Meifert, F. (1991). Berichte aus der Unwelt—Der Wiener Aktionismus und das Werk von Günter Brus als Spiegel vorgeburtlicher Erlebniswelten. In *Die kulturelle Verarbeitung pränatalen und perinatalen Erlebens,* ed. L. Janus. Heidelberg: Textstudio Gross.

Meifert, F. (1990). Zweimal Geborene–Der "Wiener Aktionismus" im Spiegel von Mythen, Riten und Gesichten. In *Protokolle*, vol. 1, ed. O. Breicha. Vienna: Jugend und Volk.

Meltzoff, A., and Moore, K. (1977). Imitation of facial and manual gestures by human neonates. *Science* 198:75–78.

Mendel, G. (1972). *Die Revolte gegen den Vater*. Frankfurt/Main: Fischer.

Meyer-Schubert, A. (1993). Weibliche Identität und fetales Selbst. *International Journal of Prenatal and Perinatal Psychology and Medicine* 5:349–360.

Mittendorfer, M. (1980). *Psychologie der pränatalen Zeit*. Salzburg: Institut für Psychologie.

Mott, F. (1964). *The Universal Design of Creation*. Edenbridge: Mark Beech.

Müller, D. (1973). *Die subakuten Massenverschiebungen des Gehirns unter der Geburt*. (*Displacement of the Brain during Birth*) Stuttgart: Thieme.

———— (1989). Personal communication.

———— (1990a). Natürlichkeitsbestrebungen und naturwissenschaftliche Realitäten im Zusammenhang mit Schwangerschaft und Geburt. In *Perinatale Medizin*, ed. J. Dudenhausen and E. Saling. Stuttgart: Thieme.

———— (1990b). Natural birth—hope and reality. *Triangle* 29:189–204.

———— (1991). Die Zwangsläufigkeit des Geburtstraumas als Folge der Evolutionspathologie des Menschen. In *Die kulturelle Verarbeitung pränatalen und perinatalen Erlebens*, ed. L. Janus. Heidelberg: Textstudio Gross.

Mureck, C. (1990). Die Hölle ist da, feiern wir das wärmende Feuer. *Konkursbuch* 25. Tübingen: Claudia Gehrke.

Murphy, G., and Wetzel, R. (1980). Suicide risk by birth, cohort in the United States, 1949 to 1974. *Archives of General Psychiatry* 37:519–523.

Murray, M. (1930). The bundle of life. In *Ancient Egypt*, ed. F. Petrie, pp. 65–73. London: Macmillan.

Naaktgeboren, C., and Slijper, E. (1970). *Biologie der Geburt.* Berlin: Paul Parey.

Neumann, E. (1956). *Die Gorße Mutter.* Zurich: Rhein Verlag. (*The Great Mother: An Analysis of the Archetype.* Princeton, NJ: Princeton University Press, 1964.)

Niemitz, C., ed. (1987). *Erbe und Umwelt.* Frankfurt/Main: Suhrkamp.

Nissen, G., ed. (1982). *Psychiatrie des Säuglings—und Kleinkindalters.* Bern: Huber.

Noble, E. (1993). *Primal Connections: How Our Experiences from Conception to Birth Influence Our Emotions, Behavior and Health.* New York: Simon & Schuster.

Nunberg, H., and Federn, E. (1962). *Minutes of the Vienna Psychoanalytic Society.* New York: International Universities Press.

Odent, M. (1986). *Von Geburt an gesund.* Munich: Kösel.

———— (1988). From psychoneuroendocrinology to primal health: new concepts as strategic tools. In *Prenatal and Perinatal Psychology and Medicine,* ed. P. Fedor-Freybergh and V. Vogel. Casterton Hall: Parthenon.

Odermatt, L. S. (1987). Aspekte der Magersucht in Bildern der Märchensprache. *Kind und Umwelt* 53:24–49.

Olschak, B. C. (1974). Bewußtwerdung unbewußter Inhalte in der fernöstlichen Psychologie. In *Pränatale Psychologie,* ed. G. H. Graber. Munich: Kindler.

Orban, P. (1980). Disco. *Kindheit* 2:1–16.

Orr, L., and Ray, S. (1977). *Rebirthing in the New Age.* Millbrae: Celestial Arts.

Pahlen, K. (1981). *Die Zauberflöte.* Munich: Goldmann.

Papousek, H. (1979). Verhaltensweisen der Mutter und des Neugeborenen unmittelbar nach der Geburt. *Archives of Gynecology* 228:1–4.

Parncutt, R. (1993). Prenatal experience and the origins of music. In *Prenatal Perceptions, Learning and Bonding,* ed. T. Blum. Heidelberg: Textstudio Gross.

Pasamanick, B., and Knobloch, H. (1966). Retrospective studies on the epidemiology of reproductive casuality: old and new. *Merrill Palmer Quarterly* 12:7–26.

Pavlov, J. P. (1955). *Sämtliche Werke, Vol. III.* Berlin: Akademie-Verlag.

Pearce, J. (1978). *Die magische Welt des Kindes.* Munich: Diederichs. (*Magical Child.* New York: Bantam, 1981.)

Peters, D. (1988). Maternal stress increases fetal brain and neonatal cerebral cortex 5-hydroxy-tryptamine synthesis in rats: a possible mechanism by which stress influences brain development. *Pharmacology, Biochemistry and Behaviour* 35:943–947.

Petrie, F., ed. (1930). *Ancient Egypt.* London: Macmillan.

Pfortenbuch, Das. (1984). In *Ägyptische Unterweltsbücher,* ed. E. Hornung. Zurich: Artemis.

Piontelli, A. (1987). Infant observation from before the birth. *International Review of Psycho-Analysis* 16:413–426.

Plaut, A. (1959). Historical and cultural aspects of the uterus. *Annals of the New York Academy of Science* 75:389–411.

Portmann, A. (1969). *Biologische Fragmente zu einer Lehre vom Menschen.* Basel: Schwabe.

Prechtl, H. (1987). Wie entwickelt sich das Verhalten vor der Geburt? In *Erbe und Umwelt,* ed. C. Niemitz. Frankfurt/Main: Suhrkamp.

Propp, V. (1975). *Die Morphologie des Märchens.* Frankfurt/Main: Suhrkamp. (*Morphology of the Folktale.* Austin, TX: University of Texas Press, 1968.)

——— (1987). *Die Wurzel des Zaubermärchens.* Munich: Hanser. (*Theory and History of Folklore.* Minneapolis, MN: University of Minnesota Press, 1984.)

Raffai, J. (1991). Auf dem Weg zur neuen somatopsychoanalytischen Therapie der Schizophrenie. In *Erscheinungsweisen pränatalen und perinatalen Erlebens in den psychotherapeutischen Settings,* ed. L. Janus. Heidelberg: Textstudio Gross.

——— (1995). The psychoanalysis of somatic sensations: the prenatal roots of schizophrenia. *International Journal of Prenatal and Perinatal Psychology and Medicine* 7:39–42.

———— (1996). The intrauterine mother representation. *International Journal of Prenatal and Perinatal Psychology and Medicine* 8:357–365.

Raikov, V. (1980). Age regression to infancy by adult subjects in deep hypnosis. *American Journal of Clinical Hypnosis* 22:156–163.

Rank, O. (1909). *Der Mythos von der Geburt des Helden*. Leipzig and Vienna: Deuticke. (*The Myth of the Birth of the Hero:* New York: Vintage, 1959.)

———— (1924). *Das Trauma der Geburt*. Frankfurt/Main: Fischer, 1988 (*The Trauma of Birth*. New York: Dover, 1993.)

———— (1926). *Die analytische Situation. Technik der Psychoanalyse, Vol. I*. Leipzig: Deuticke.

Rank, O., and Sachs, H. (1965). *Die Bedeutung der Psychoanalyse für die Geisteswissenschaften*. Amsterdam: Bonset.

Ranke-Graves, R. (1985). *Griechische Mythologie*. Reinbek: Rowohlt.

Raphael-Leff, J. (1991). *Psychological Processes of Childbearing*. London: Chapman and Hall.

Ratner, A. (1991). Spätfolgen geburtstraumatischer Läsionen des zentralen Nervensystems. *Der Kinderarzt* 22:385–391.

Rauchfleisch, U. (1981). *Dissozial*. Göttingen: Vandenhoeck und Ruprecht.

Rausch, H. (1988a). Die "Epileptische Reaktion" als Extrembeispiel eines psychosomatischen Geschehens prä- und perinatale Aspekte. In *Das Leben vor und während der Geburt*, ed. G. Schusser and W. Hartzmann. Osnabrück: Universitätsdruck Osnabrück.

Rausch, H. (1988b). Das psychotische Geschehen im Lichte der prä- und perinatalen Psychologie. Ref. 19. Internationale Symposium der Deutschen Akademie für Psychoanalyse. Unpublished manuscript.

———— (1991). Biologische und psychosoziale Aspekte der kulturellen Evolution. In *Die kulturelle Verarbeitung pränatalen und perinatalen Erlebens*. Heidelberg: Textstudio Gross.

Reinold, E. (1982). Das vorgeburtliche Verhalten des Feten aus der

Sicht des Geburtshelfers. In *Pränatale und Perinatale Psychosomatik*, ed. T. Hau and S. Schindler. Stuttgart: Hippokrates.

Reiter, A. (1995). Pränatale Wurzeln Phobischer Ängste. *International Journal of Prenatal and Perinatal Psychology and Medicine* 7:509–528.

Rice, R. (1986). The mind–body connection: ancient and modern healing strategies for a a traumatic birth and the sick newborn. *Pre- and Perinatal Psychology* 1:11–19.

Riedl, R. (1985). *Die Spaltung des Weltbildes.* Berlin: Paul Parey.

Roebling, I. (1985). Prinzip Heimat—eine regressive Utopie? In *Schriften der Theodor-Storm-Gesellschaft* 34. Heide: Verlagsanstalt Boyens.

———— (1990). Uber prä- und perinatale Phantasien in der neuzeitlichen bürgerlichen Gesellschaft. In *Das Seelenleben der Ungeborenen—eine Wurzel unseres Unbewußten*, ed. L. Janus. Pfaffenweiler: Centaurus.

Röd, W. (1962). *Descartes.* Munich: Reinhardt.

Rosen, D. (1975). Suicide survivors: a follow-up study of persons who survived jumping from the Golden Gate and San Francisco-Oakland Bay bridges. *Western Journal of Medicine* 122:289ff.

Rotter, F. (1985). *Musik als Kommunikationsmedium.* Berlin: Duncker und Humboldt.

Rottmann, G. (1974). Untersuchungen über die Einstellung zur Schwangerschaft und zur Fötalen Entwicklung. In *Pränatale Psychologie*, ed. G. H. Graber. Munich: Kindler.

Ryder, G. (1943). Vagitus Uterinus. *American Journal of Obstetrics and Gynecology* 46:867–872.

Sachs, N. (1961). *Fahrt ins Staublose. Die Gedichte der Nelly Sachs.* Frankfurt/Main: Suhrkamp.

Saenger, H. (1924). Uber die Entstehung intrakranieller Blutungen beim Neugeborenen. *Monatsschrift für Geburtshilfe und Gynäkologie* 65:257–274.

Sahlberg, O. (1986). *Rausch und Realität: Die Aktualitat Gottfried Benns.* Iserlohn: Evangelische Akademie.

—— (1991). Die Heilung des Geburtstraumas im Werk Gottfried Benns. In *Die kulturelle Verarbeitung pränatalen und perinatalen Erlebens*, ed. L. Janus. Heidelberg: Textstudio Gross.

Salk, L. (1973). The role of the heartbeat in the relations between mother and infant. *Scientific American* 228:24–29.

—— (1974). Perinatal complications in the history of the asthmatic. *Children—American Journal of Diseases of Children* 127:30–33.

—— (1985). Relationship of maternal and perinatal conditions to eventual adolescent suicide. *Lancet* 1:624–627.

Schachtinger, H. (1987). Verhaltensausstattung und erste Anpassungsleistungen. In *Erbe und Umwelt*, ed. C. Niemitz. Frankfurt/Main: Suhrkamp.

Schepank, H. (1987). *Psychogene Erkrankungen der Stadtbevölkerung.* (*Epidemiology of Psychogenic Disorders*) Heidelberg: Springer.

Scherf, W. (1972). *Lexikon der Zaubermärchen.* Stuttgart: Diederichs.

Schier, K. (1993). The analysis of appearance and meaning of prenatal and perinatal phantasies in the psychoanalytically oriented psychotherapy of children. *International Journal of Prenatal and Perinatal Psychology and Medicine* 5:433–438.

Schilder, P. (1973). *Entwurf zu einer Psychiatrie auf psychoanalytischer Grundlage.* Frankfurt/Main: Suhrkamp.

Schiller, F. (1982). *Sämtliche Werke, Vol. I.* Munich: Hanser.

Schindler, S., ed. (1982). *Geburt—Entritt in eine neue Welt.* Göttingen: Hogrefe.

—— (1984). Zur Situation des Kindes in der Schwangerschaft und Geburt—Aspekte der pränatalen Psychologie. *Tutzinger Materialien* 13:21.

—— (1983). Was bedeutet die Einbeziehung der pränatalen Zeit für die Psychoanalyse. In *Psychoanalyse Heute, Revision oder Re-Vision Freuds?*, ed. R. Larcher. Vienna: Literas.

Schindler, S., and Zimprich, H., eds. (1983). *Ökologie der Perinatalzeit.* Stuttgart: Hippokrates.

Schusser, G., and Hatzmann, W. (1988). *Das Leben vor und während der Geburt.* Osnabrück: *Universitätsdruck Osnabrück.*

Schwartz, L. (1983). Die Welt des ungeborenen Kindes. In *Psychedelic Reflections*, ed. L. Grinspoon and J. B. Bakalar. New York: Human Sciences.

Schwartz, P. (1964). *Geburtsschäden bei Neugeborenen*. Jena: Gustav Fischer.

———— (1968). Die Geburtsschädigung des Gehirns Neugeborener. *Deutsches Ärzteblatt* 43:2383–2390.

Secrest, M. (1987). *Salvador Dalí*. Bern and Munich: Schirmer/ Mosel.

Selye, H. (1974). *Streß*. Munich: Piper. (*The Stress of Life*. New York: McGraw-Hill, 1978.)

Sendak, M. (1987). *Wo die wilden Kerle wohnen*. (*Where the Wild Things Are*) Zurich: Diogenes.

Share, L. (1994). *If Someone Speaks, It Gets Lighter*. Hillsdale, NJ: Analytic Press.

———— (1996). Dreams and the reconstruction of the infant trauma. *International Journal of Prenatal and Perinatal Psychology and Medicine* 8:295–316.

Simon, A. (1988). *Beckett*. Frankfurt/Main: Suhrkamp.

Sloterdijk, P. (1986). 10 kleine, teils freche, teils begründete Bemerkungen zum Komplex Philosophie, Psychologie und Existenz. *Gruppentherapie und Gruppendynamik* 22:257–258.

———— (1988). *Zur Welt kommen—Zur Sprache kommen*. Frankfurt/ Main: Suhrkamp.

———— (1993). Weltfremdheit. Frankfurt/Main: Suhrkamp.

Sollner, W., et al. (1989). *Soziopsychosomatik*. Heidelberg: Springer.

Sonne, J. C. (1994a). The relevance of the dread of being aborted to models of therapy and models of the mind: part I: case examples. *International Journal of Prenatal and Perinatal Psychology and Medicine* 6:67–86.

———— (1994b). The relevance of the dread of being aborted to models of therapy and models of the mind: part II; mentation and communication with the unborn. *International Journal of Prenatal and Perinatal Psychology and Medicine* 6:247–275.

———— (1996). Interpreting the dread of being aborted in therapy.

International Journal of Prenatal and Perinatal Psychology and Medicine 8:317–339.

Sontag, L. (1944). War and the fetal-maternal relationship. *Journal of Marriage and the Family* 6:3–16.

——— (1966). Implications of fetal behavior and environment of adult personalities. *Annals of the New York Academy of Science* 134:762–768.

Stellberg, R. (1988). Rebirthing als transpersonale Psychotherapie. In *Das Leben vor und während der Geburt*, ed. G. Schusser and W. Hatzmann. Osnabrück: Universitätsdruck Osnabrück.

Sternberg, L. (1930). Der Adlerkult bei den Völkern Sibiriens. *Archiv für Religionswissenschaften* 28:125–153.

Stifter, A. (1959). *Gesammelte Werke*, vol. 6. Sigbert Mohn.

Stirnimann, F. (1940). *Psychologie des neugeborenen Kindes*. Munich: Kindler.

Storch, R. (1991). Experience from psychotherapeutic treatment of prematurely born children. *International Journal of Prenatal and Perinatal Studies* 3:125–130.

Storm, T. (1982). Die Regentrude. *Sämtliche Werke, Vol. I.* Munich: Winkler.

Stott, D. (1973). Follow-up study from birth of the effects of prenatal stresses. *Developmental Medicine and Child Neurology* 15: 770–778.

Strasser, W. (1988). *Heilen mit Lebensenergie*. Munich: Psychologische Fachbuchhandlung.

Strauss, M. (1983). *Von der Zeichensprache des kleinen Kindes*. Stuttgart: Freies Geistesleben.

Strobel, W. (1991). Aktualisierung prä- und perinatalen Erlebens und korrigierende Neuerfahrungen in der klanggeleiteten Trance. In *Erscheinungsweisen prä- und perinatalen Erlebens in den psychotherapeutischen Settings*, ed. L. Janus. Heidelberg: Textstudio Gross.

Süskind, P. (1985). *Das Parfum*. Zurich: Diogenes. (*Perfume: The Story of a Murderer*. New York: Knopf, 1986.)

Telerent, A., et al. (1991). Prenatal and perinatal memories collected from psychotic adolescents. *International Journal of Prenatal and Perinatal Studies* 3:169–174.

Terr, L. C. (1991). Childhood traumas: an outline and overview. *American Journal of Psychiatry* 148:10–20.

Theweleit, K. (1977). *Männerphantasien.* Frankfurt/Main: Stroemfeld. (*Male Fantasies*, vols. 1 and 2. Minneapolis, MN: University of Minnesota Press, 1987, 1989.)

Thomson, W. R. (1957). Influence of prenatal maternal anxiety on emotionality in young rats. *Science* 125:698.

Tomatis, A. (1987). *Der Klang des Lebens.* Reinbeck: Rowohlt.

Trevathan, W. (1990). The evolution of helplessness in the human infant and its significance for pre- and perinatal psychology. *Pre- and Perinatal Psychology* 4:267–280.

Tronick, E., and Adamson, L. (1980). *Babies as People: New Findings on Our Social Beginnings.* New York: Collier.

Truby, H., Bosma, J. F., and Lind, J. (1965). The newborn infant cry. *Acta Paediatrica Scandinavica* 163, suppl.

Trunz, E. (1967). Anmerkungen des Herausgebers. In *Goethes Werke*, vol. 2. Hamburg: Wegener.

Turnbull, C. (1983). *The Human Cycle.* New York: Simon & Schuster.

van der Kolk, B. (1987). *Psychological Trauma.* Washington, DC: American Psychiatric Press.

Veldman, F. (1988). *Haptonomie—Science de l'Affectivité.* Paris: Presses Universitaires de France.

——— (1991). Haptonomie—Wissenschaft von den Grundlagen der Affektivität. In *Erscheinungsweisen pränatalen und perinatalen Erlebens in den psychotherapeutischen Settings*, ed. L. Janus, pp. 15–31. Heidelberg: Textstudio Gross.

——— (1994). Confirming affectivity in the dawn of life. *International Journal of Prenatal and Perinatal Psychology and Medicine* 6:11–26.

Verny, T., and Kelly, J. (1983). *Das Seelenleben des Ungeborenen.* Frankfurt/Main: Ullstein. (*The Secret Life of the Unborn Child.* New York: Delacorte, 1982.)

Verny, T., and Weintraub, P. (1992). *Das Leben vor der Gerburt. Ein Neun-Monate Programm für Sie und Ihr Ungeborenes.* Frankfurt: Zeitausendeins. (*Nurturing the Unborn Child.* New York: Delacorte, 1991.)

Ward, I., and Ward, B. (1989). Reproductive behavior and physiology in prenatally stressed males. In *Frontiers in Stress Research,* ed. H. Weiner. Bern: Huber.

Wasdell, D. (1991a). Das Geburtstrauma und die Dynamik der globalen politischen Entwicklung. In *Die kulturelle Verarbeitung pränatalen und perinatalen Erlebens,* ed. L. Janus. Heidelberg: Textstudio Gross.

——— (1991b). Prä- und perinatale Grundlagen der soziopolitischen Dynamik. In *Erscheinungsweisen pränatalen und perinatalen Erlebens in den psychotherapeutischen Settings,* ed. L. Janus. Heidelberg: Textstudio Gross.

——— (1993). *Die pränatalen und perinatalen Wurzeln von Religion und Krieg.* Pfaffenweiler: Centaurus.

——— (1994). Mary findet wieder Anschlußs an sich selbst. In *Ungewollte Kinder,* ed. H. Häsing and L. Janus. Reinbek: Rowohlt.

——— (1995). Birth time and the dynamics of social systems. *International Journal of Prenatal and Perinatal Psychology and Medicine* 7:475–481.

Weiner, H., ed. (1989). *Frontiers in Stress Research.* Bern: Huber.

Werner, E., and Smith, R. (1982). *Vulnerable but Invincible.* New York: McGraw-Hill.

Wilber, K. (1987). *Halbzeit der Evolution.* Bern: Scherz.

Wilheim, J. (1992). The emergence of early traumatic imprints in psychoanalytic practice. *International Journal of Prenatal and Perinatal Studies* 4:179–186.

——— (1995). *Unterwegs zur Geburt.* Heidelberg: Mattes.

Winnicott, D. W. (1988). *Human Nature.* London: Free Association Press.

——— (1992). Birth memories, birth trauma and anxiety. *International Journal of Prenatal and Perinatal Studies* 4:17–34.

Wischnik, A. (1989). Neue Aspekte der radiologischen Pelvimetrie. *Zeitschrift für Geburtshilfe und Perinatologie* 193:145–151.

Zeier, H., ed. (1977). *Pawlow und die Folgen.* Zurich: Kindler.

Zeskind, P. (1978). Acoustic features and auditory perceptions of the cries of newborns with prenatal and perinatal complications. *Child Development* 49:580–589.

Prenatal Societies and Journals

There are two international societies, one American, the Association for Pre- and Perinatal Psychology and Health (APPPH), 340 Colony Road, Box 994, Geyserville, CA 95441, Tel: (707) 857–4041, Fax: (707) 857–3764, and one European, the International Society for Prenatal and Perinatal Psychology and Medicine (ISPPM), Friedhofweg 8, D-Heidelberg, Germany, Tel: +49-6221-892729, Fax: +49-6221-892730. The ISPPM was founded in 1971 at the International Psychoanalytical Congress in Vienna by the three psychoanalysts Igor Caruso, Gustav Hans Graber, and Arnaldo Rascovsky. It is interdisciplinary but also cultivates its own psychoanalytical tradition. The APPPH journal is the *Pre- and Perinatal Psychology Journal*, Human Sciences Press,

233 Spring Street, New York, New York 10013-1578, and the ISPPM-Journal is the *International Journal for Prenatal and Perinatal Psychology and Medicine,* Mattes, Johann-Fischer-Str. 6/1, D - 69121 Heidelberg. German articles have synopses in English. Both societies organize local and international conferences for scientific exchange.

Index

ABOUT THE AUTHOR

Dr. Ludwig Janus was born in Essen, Germany. He completed his studies in medicine in Munich, Essen, and Göttingen and received his psychoanalytic education in Göttingen and Heidelberg. Since 1975, Dr. Janus has been a psychoanalyst practicing in Heidelberg, and a teacher and training analyst at institutes in Heidelberg, Saarbrücken, and Frankfurt. He holds a professorship in prenatal psychology in Frankfurt. A member of several societies, notably for prenatal psychology and psychohistory, Dr. Janus has written more than 100 articles on psychoanalysis, prenatal psychology, and psychohistory, and four books on prenatal psychology. He is the editor of several books on prenatal psychology and documentaries on psychohistory.

Dr. Janus is married and has six children.